RESEARCH AND PERSPECTIVES IN ALZHEIMER'S DISEASE

Fondation Ipsen

S. R. Rapoport   H. Petit
D. Leys   Y. Christen (Eds.)

Imaging, Cerebral Topography and Alzheimer's Disease

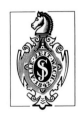

Springer-Verlag
Berlin Heidelberg New York
London Paris Tokyo Hong Kong

Rapoport, Stanley I., M.D.
Laboratory of Neurosciences
National Institute on Aging
National Institutes of Health
Bethesda, MA 20892, USA

Petit, Henri, M.D.
A.D.E.R.M.A., Faculté de Médecine
Université de Lille
1, place de Verdun
F-59045 Lille Cédex

Leys, Didier, M.D.
A.D.E.R.M.A., Faculté de Médecine
Université de Lille
1, place de Verdun
F-59045 Lille Cédex

Christen, Yves, Ph. D.
Fondation IPSEN pour la Recherche Thérapeutique,
30, rue Cambronne, F-75737 Paris Cédex

ISBN 3-540-52552-1 Springer-Verlag Berlin Heidelberg New York
ISBN 0-387-52552-1 Springer-Verlag New York Berlin Heidelberg

Library of Congress Cataloging-in-Publication Data. Imaging, cerebral topography, and Alzheimer's disease / S.I. Rapoport ... [et al.] (eds.). p. cm. — (Research and perspectives in Alzheimer's disease) ISBN 0-387-52552-1 (U.S. : alk. paper) 1. Alzheimer's disease—Imaging. 2. Brain—Imaging. I. Rapoport, Stanley I. II. Series. [DNLM: 1. Alzheimer's Disease—diagnosis. 2. Brain—pathology. 3. Diagnostic Imaging. WM 220 I31]. RC523.I46 1990 618.97′68310757—dc20 DNLM/DLC 90-9766

Typesetting, printed and bookbinding: Triltsch, Würzburg
2127/3020-543210 – Printed on acid-free paper

Preface

This volume contains the proceedings of the fifth Colloque Médecine et Recherche organized by the Fondation Ipsen pour la Recherche Thérapeutique and devoted to Alzheimer's disease. It was held in Lille on October 16, 1989 and dedicated to imaging, cerebral topography and Alzheimer's disease.

The proceedings of the previous meetings were published as the present one in the same series: *Immunology and Alzheimer's disease* (A. Pouplard-Barthelaix, J. Emile, Y. Christen eds.), *Genetics in Alzheimer's disease* (P.-M. Sinet, Y. Lamour, Y. Christen eds.) in 1988, *Neuronal grafting and Alzheimer's disease* (F. Gage, A. Privat, Y. Christen eds.), *Biological markers of Alzheimer's disease* (F. Boller, R. Katzman, A. Rascol, J.-L. Signoret, Y. Christen eds.) in 1989.

The next meeting of the series entitled *growth factors and Alzheimer's disease* was being held in Strasbourg on April 25, 1990. The proceedings will be published by the end of this year.

Yves Christen
Vice-Président of the Fondation Ipsen pour la Recherche Thérapeutique

Acknowledgements: The editors wish to express their gratitude to Y. Lamour (Paris), A. Syrota (Paris), J. Clarisse (Lille), F. Boller (Paris), C. Manelfe (Toulouse) and M. Steinling (Lille) for their collaboration as chairmen for the meeting, Mary Lynn Gage for her editorial assistance and Jacqueline Mervaillie for the organization of the meeting.

Contents

Contributors

Agniel, A.
INSERM U. 230 et Service de Neurologie, CHU Purpan, 31059 Toulouse
Cédex, France

Baron, J. C.
INSERM U. 320 and Cyceron B.P. 5027, 14021 Caen Cédex, France

Bouras, C.
Département de Psychiatrie, IUPG Bel Air, Université de Genève,
1225 Chêne-Bourg, Geneva, Switzerland

Bowen, D. M.
Miriam Marks Department of Neurochemistry, Institute of Neurology
(Queen Square), 1, Wakefield Street, London WC1N 1PJ, UK

Campbell, M. J.
Fishberg Research Center for Neurobiology and Department of Geriatrics
and Adult Development, Box 1065, Mount Sinai School of Medicine,
One Gustave L. Levy Place, New York, NY 10029, USA

Celsis, P.
INSERM U. 230 et Service de Neurologie, CHU Purpan, 31059 Toulouse
Cédex, France

Clarisse, J.
Departments of Neuroradiology, Université de Lille, Faculté de Médecine,
1 place de Verdun, 59045 Lille Cédex, France

Cox, K.
Department of Neurosciences, University of California, School of Medicine
San Diego, La Jolla, CA 92093, USA

Creasey, H.
Department of Geriatric Medicine, University of Sydney, Concord RG
Hospital, Concord 2139, Australia

Cross, A. J.
Astra Neuroscience Research Unit, Institute of Neurology (Queen Square), 1, Wakefield Street, London WC1N 1PJ, UK

Défossez, A.
Laboratories of Histology (INSERM U. 156), Université de Lille, Faculté de Médecine, 1 place de Verdun, 59045 Lille Cédex, France

Delacourte, A.
Laboratories of Neurosciences (INSERM U. 16), Université de Lille, Faculté de Médecine, 1 place de Verdun, 59045 Lille Cédex, France

Delaère, P.
Laboratoire de Neuropathologie R. Escourolle, FRA Association Claude Bernard, Hôpital de La Salpêtrière, 47 bd de l'Hôpital, 75651 Paris Cédex 13, France

De Lima, A. D.
Max-Planck-Institut für Entwicklungsbiologie, Spemannstraße 35/I, 7400 Tübingen, FRG

Démonet, J. F.
INSERM U. 230 et Service de Neurologie, CHU Purpan, 31059 Toulouse Cédex, France

Duyckaerts, C.
Laboratoire de Neuropathologie R. Escourolle, FRA Association Claude Bernard, Hôpital de La Salpêtrière, 47 bd de l'Hôpital, 75651 Paris Cédex 13, France

Frackowiak, R. S. J.
National Hospital, Queen Square and MRC Cyclotron Unit, Royal Postgraduate Medical School, London, UK

Francis, P. T.
Miriam Marks Departments of Neurochemistry, Institute of Neurology (Queen Square), 1, Wakefield Street, London WC1N 1PJ, UK

Grady, C. L.
Laboratory of Neurosciences, National Institute on Aging, Bldg 10, Room 6C414, National Institutes of Health, Bethesda, MD 20892, USA

Green, A. R.
Astra Neuroscience Research Unit, Institute of Neurology (Queen Square), 1, Wakefield Street, London WC1N 1PJ, UK

Hauw, J.-J.
Laboratoire de Neuropathologie R. Escourolle, FRA Association Claude
Bernard, Hôpital de La Salpêtrière, 47 bd de l'Hôpital, 75651 Paris
Cédex 13, France

Haxby, J. V.
Laboratory of Neurosciences, National Institute on Aging, Bldg 10,
Room 6C414, National Institutes of Health, Bethesda, MD 20892, USA

Hof, P. R.
Fishberg Research Center for Neurobiology and Department of Geriatrics
and Adult Development, Box 1065, Mount Sinai School of Medicine,
One Gustave L. Levy Place, New York, NY 10029, USA

Klunk, W. E.
University of Pittsburgh, Western Psychiatric Institute and Clinic,
The Graduate School of Public Health, 130 DeSoto St., Crabtree Hall,
Pittsburgh, PA 15261, USA

Lassen, N. A.
Department of Neurology, Rigshospitalet, 9, Blegdamsvej,
2100 Copenhagen, Denmark

Leys, D.
Departments of Neurology, Université de Lille, Faculté de Médecine,
1 place de Verdun, 59045 Lille Cédex, France

Lowe, S. L.
Miriam Marks Department of Neurochemistry, Institute of Neurology
(Queen Square), 1, Wakefield Street, London WC1N 1PJ, UK

Luxenberg, J.
Laboratory of Neurosciences, National Institute on Aging, National
Institutes of Health, Bethesda, MD 20892, USA

Marc-Vergnes, J. P.
INSERM U. 230 et Service de Neurologie, CHU Purpan, 31059 Toulouse
Cédex, France

Morrison, J. H.
Fishberg Research Center for Neurobiology and Department of Geriatrics
and Adult Development, Box 1065, Mount Sinai School of Medicine,
One Gustave L. Levy Place, New York, NY 10029, USA

Parent, M.
Laboratories of Neuropathology, Université de Lille, Faculté de Médecine,
1 place de Verdun, 59045 Lille Cédex, France

Paulson, O. B.
Department of Neurology, Rigshospitalet, 9, Blegdamsvej,
2100 Copenhagen, Denmark

Petit, H.
Departments of Neurology, Université de Lille, Faculté de Médecine,
1 place de Verdun, 59045 Lille Cédex, France

Pettegrew, J. W.
University of Pittsburgh, Western Psychiatric Institute and Clinic,
The Graduate School of Public Health, 130 DeSoto St., Crabtree Hall,
Pittsburgh, PA 15261, USA

Piette, F.
Hôpital Charles Foix, 7, avenue de la République, 94205 Ivry/Seine, France

Procter, A. W.
Miriam Marks Department of Neurochemistry, Institute of Neurology
(Queen Square), 1, Wakefield Street, London WC1N 1PJ, UK

Pruvo, J.-P.
Departments of Neuroradiology, Université de Lille, Faculté de Médecine,
1 place de Verdun, 59045 Lille Cédex, France

Puel, M.
INSERM U. 230 et Service de Neurologie, CHU Purpan, 31059 Toulóuse
Cédex, France

Rapoport, A.
Departments of Neurology, Université de Lille, Faculté de Médecine,
1 place de Verdun, 59045 Lille Cédex, France

Rapoport, S. I.
Laboratory of Neurosciences, National Institute on Aging, National
Institutes of Health, Bethesda, MD 20892, USA

Rascol, A.
INSERM U. 230 et Service de Neurologie, CHU Purpan, 31059 Toulouse
Cédex, France

Rossor, M. N.
National Hospital, Queen Square and MRC Cyclotron Unit,
Royal Postgraduate Medical School, London, UK

Schapiro, M.
Laboratory of Neurosciences, National Institute on Aging, Bldg 10,
Room 6C414, National Institutes of Health, Bethesda, MD 20892, USA

Soetaert, G.
Katholiek Universiteit Leuven, Leuven, Belgium

Steele, J. E.
Miriam Marks Department of Neurochemistry, Institute of Neurology
(Queen Square), 1, Wakefield Street, London WC1N 1PJ, UK

Steinling, M.
NMR Imaging, Hôpital B. Lille, 1 place de Verdun, 59037 Lille Cédex,
France

Stratmann, G. C.
Miriam Marks Department of Neurochemistry, Institute of Neurology
(Queen Square), 1, Wakefield Street, London WC1N 1PJ, UK

Tyrrell, P.J.
National Hospital, Queen Square and MRC Cyclotron Unit,
Royal Postgraduate Medical School, London, UK

Vermersch, P.
Departments of Neurology, Université de Lille, Faculté de Médecine,
1 place de Verdun, 59045 Lille Cédex, France

Voigt, T.
Max-Planck-Institut für Entwicklungsbiologie, Spemannstraße 35/I,
7400 Tübingen, FRG

Waldemar, G.
Department of Neurology, Rigshospitalet, 9, Blegdamsvej,
2100 Copenhagen, Denmark

Young, W. G.
Department of Neuropharmacology, Research Institute of Scripps Clinic,
BCR-1, 10666 North Torrey Pines Road, La Jolla, CA 92037, USA

Topography of Alzheimer's Disease: Involvement of Association Neocortices and Connected Regions; Pathological, Metabolic and Cognitive Correlations; Relation to Evolution

S. I. Rapoport

Summary

Alzheimer's disease (AD) patients display reduced glucose metabolism and increased right-left metabolic asymmetries in the association neocortices early and throughout the clinical course, with relative sparing of primary sensory and motor neocortical regions. The metabolic asymmetries precede and predict neocortically mediated cognitive deficits. They also correspond with the distribution of AD neuropathology in the association, as compared with primary sensory and motor, neocortices. Outside of the neocortex, pathology is distributed mainly in brain regions functionally and anatomically connected with the association neocortex – medial septal nucleus, nucleus basalis of Meynert, CA1 and subicular subfields of hippocampal formation, layers II and IV of entorhinal cortex, corticobasal nuclear group of amygdaloid formation, cortically projecting neurons of the dorsal raphe and locus coeruleus. Comparative anatomical studies suggest that many of these regions evolved disproportionately in higher primates, particularly in hominids, by a process termed "integrative phylogeny." Thus, the topographic distribution of functional and pathological abnormalities in AD suggests that AD is a phylogenic disease. Regional vulnerability to the disease may have been introduced into the primate genome during evolution, possibly by regulatory mutations. The topographic correspondence of neuropathology and functional deficits in AD and demented adults with Down's syndrome suggests, furthermore, that a genomic change equivalent to increased expression of genes on human chromosome 21 introduced the AD process during evolution.

Why Determine the Topography of Neurodegenerative Disorders?

In the last decade, it has become possible to examine the topography of certain human neurodegenerative diseases by means of positron emission tomography (PET), early and throughout their clinical course (Huang et al. 1980). For example, with an appropriate positron emitting isotope, such as [^{18}F]2-fluoro-2-deoxy-D-glucose (^{18}FDG), and a sensitive PET scanner, we can now examine regional cerebral metabolic rates for glucose ($rCMR_{glc}$) within areas of the human brain as small as 6 mm in diameter, on the cortical surface as well as subcortically

(Grady et al. 1989 a). As glucose is the major substrate for brain oxidative metabolism, its rate of consumption is a direct measure of regional brain functional activity.

Positron emission tomography studies during life, if consistent with postmortem neuropathology and neurochemistry, make it easier to guess which brain regions are initially affected in a given disorder, and which degenerate in a secondary manner. This is important because postmortem studies alone cannot identify the order of pathological events, but only the final picture. By using PET to ascertain which brain regions are affected early in the course of a disease, it should be possible to generate hypotheses and experimental approaches to better understand its pathogenesis, with regard to factors such as genetics, environmental exposure, regional connectivity, or regional metabolic, molecular biological or neurotransmitter differences. Furthermore, because man is an animal who reached his present form through genetic mutation, natural selection and adaptation to changing environments (Darwin 1871), regional differences in disease vulnerability can also be considered in terms of evolutionary principles (Hughlings Jackson 1884; Roofe and Matzky 1968; Rapoport 1988 a, b, 1989).

Comparative anatomical data suggest that the brain not only increased in size during recent primate evolution but also underwent disproportionate expansion and differentiation of certain systems of related regions (cf. Luria 1973) according to the principle of "integrated phylogeny" (Rapoport 1988 a, 1989, in preparation). Furthermore, human neurological disorders may affect such systems according to the recency of their evolutionary modifications during primate (and particularly hominid) evolution (cf. Hughlings Jackson 1884). In such cases, a neurological disease can be rightly termed "phylogenic" (Roofe and Matzke 1968; Sarnat and Netsky 1981; Rapoport 1989).

Integrative Phylogeny of Association Brain Regions

It has been proposed that several systems or ensembles of functionally and anatomically connected brain regions underwent integrated phylogeny during recent evolution of primates, particularly of hominids (Rapoport, in preparation). As illustrated in Table 1, System I regions include the association neocortices and non-neocortical telencephalic regions within the hippocampal formation (CA1 and subicular subfields), entorhinal cortex (layers II and IV), amygdaloid complex [corticobasolateral nuclear group, as defined by Stephan and Andy (1977)], nucleus basalis of Meynert and medial septal nucleus. System II regions include several frontal cortical regions, as well as parts of the thalamus, basal ganglia and substantia nigra which constitute segregated circuits contributing to motor movements and motor-related memory and other cognitive abilities (Alexander et al. 1986; Rapoport, in preparation). System III regions include the neodentate nucleus of the cerebellum, and certain neurons of pontine and mesencephalic nuclei. In general, many of the non-neocortical brain regions and their subdivisions, which expanded or differentiated disproportionately during primate evolution, are anatomically and functionally related to the association neocortices (Rapoport 1988 a,b; 1989, in preparation).

Table 1. Progression studies of telencephalic brain regions in higher primates[a]

Brain region	PI[b] man	Division with maximal progression during primate evolution
System I[c]: Telencephalic regions, including amygdala and hippocampal formation		

Neocortex	156	Association areas, including
		  Prefrontal cortex
		  Visual association
		  Broca's speech area (44 and 45, Brodman)
		  Inferior parietal lobule (39 and 40, Brodman)
		  Brodman area 37
		    (part of Wernicke's speech area)

Corpus callosum	↑	
Amygdaloid complex	3.9	Corticobasolateral group
Hippocampal formation	4.2	Subiculum, CA1 regions
Entorhinal cortex	5.5	
Septum	4.0	
Nucleus basalis of Meynert	↑	

[a] Data summarized by Rapoport (in preparation) from Stephan and Andy (1970, 1977), Stephan et al. (1970, 1987), Andy and Stephan (1966) and Gorry (1963)
[b] PI, progression index in *Homo sapiens* (ratio of weight of human brain to weight of brain in insectivore of equivalent body weight). ↑, PI > 1 but value not known in man
[c] See text for details

Several human neurological disorders probably involve brain regions of System II. These include obsessive compulsive disorder (in which metabolic abnormalities are localized in the orbitofrontal cortex, anterior cingulate gyrus, prefrontal cortex and caudate nucleus, and where the anatomy of the caudate nucleus is abnormal) (Baxter et al. 1987; Luxenberg et al. 1988; Wise and Rapoport 1988; Swedo et al. 1989), Huntington's disease (in which the caudate nucleus degenerates), and Parkinson's disease (with pathology in the substantia nigra and caudate nucleus) (Heindel et al. 1989; Rapoport, in preparation).

On the other hand, System I regions appear to be preferentially involved in Alzheimer's disease (AD), Pick's disease and Down's syndrome (Rapoport 1988 a, b, 1989; Haxby et al., this volume; Schapiro et al., 1986 and this volume). In this paper, I summarize neuropathological, PET and cognitive data which .argue for System I regional predilection to AD, and in turn suggest that AD is a human phylogenic disease. This latter interpretation implies, I believe, that understanding the genetic basis of evolution of the human brain, and particularly of AD-vulnerable regions, may elucidate the genetic basis of AD.

Neuropathology of Association Regions in the Alzheimer Brain

Abundant senile (neuritic) plaques, neurofibrillary tangles with paired helical filaments, and neuronal dropout characterize the AD brain (Terry and Wisniewski 1972; Ball and Nuttall 1981; Ball et al. 1985; Arendt et al. 1985). This

Table 2. Brain regions affected by Alzheimer pathology[a]

Association neocortices much more than primary motor or sensory neocortices
    Neurofibrillary tangles in pyramidal neurons of layers III and V; cell loss
Non-neocortical regions connected with association neocortices
    Posterior cingulate gyrus
    Entorhinal cortex (layers II and IV)
    Hippocampal formation (subiculum, CA 1 pyramidal field, dentate gyrus)
    Amygdaloid formation, corticobasal group
    Cholinergic nucleus basalis of Meynert (Ch 4)
    Medial septal nucleus (Ch 1)
    Locus coeruleus, noradrenergic cortically projecting neurons
    Dorsal raphe, serotonergic cortically projecting neurons

---

[a] See text for references

Table 3. Distribution of neurofibrillary tangles in cortical visual regions of patients with AD[a]

Age (years)	Cortical region[b]		
	17	18	20
82	0.2 ± 0.1	9.8 ± 1.5	7.8 ± 1.1
74	0.1 ± 0.1	13.0 ± 0.7	24.4 ± 1.6
71	0.1 ± 0.1	15.0 ± 1.5	22.1 ± 1.3
68	0.5 ± 0.3	19.9 ± 2.2	57.5 ± 3.9
63	2.0 ± 0.6	30.3 ± 1.6	63.5 ± 5.2
62	2.4 ± 0.5	30.4 ± 2.3	37.5 ± 2.0
Mean	$0.9 \pm 1.0*$	$19.7 \pm 3.6**$	$35.5 \pm 8.8***$

[a] Data from Lewis et al. (1987)
[b] Values for each case are the mean $\pm$ SE number of tangles in a 250-μm-wide cortical traverse from ten sections. Values not sharing same superscript are significantly different from each of the others ($p < 0.05$)

neuropathology is more severe in System I regions than in System II or other nonassociation brain regions (Table 2) (Rapoport 1988 b, in preparation). Thus, the association neocortices are more severely pathological than are primary sensory and motor regions (Brun and Gustafson 1976; Pearson et al., 1985). Although senile plaques are commonly found throughout the neocortex, neurofibrillary tangles are more common within large pyramidal neurons of layers III and V of association than of primary sensory and motor areas, as illustrated, for example, for visual regions (Table 3) (Pearson et al. 1985; Rogers and Morrison 1985; Lewis et al. 1987). Layer III and V neurons are the source of corticocortical fibers, whereas layer V neurons also give rise to corticofugal fibers (Wise and Jones 1977), and their involvement indicates disorganization of long cortical-cortical and corticofugal connections (Horwitz et al. 1987; Morrison, this volume).

Outside of the neocortex, neurofibrillary tangles are found in neurons which are closely connected, directly or indirectly, with the association neocortex, and belong mainly to the System I regions which underwent integrated phylogeny (Table 1). These cells are in layers II and IV of the entorhinal cortex, and in the subiculum, CA1 subfield and outer two-thirds of the molecular layer of the dentate gyrus of the hippocampal formation (Ball and Nuttall 1981; Kemper 1984; Hyman et al. 1984, 1986). The subiculum and entorhinal cortex connect the hippocampal formation reciprocally with the association neocortices, and their pathology in AD may functionally disconnect the hippocampal formation from these regions (Hyman et al. 1984).

Cell loss and neuropathology are also found in the posterior cingulate gyrus (Brun and Gustafson 1976), which has important connections with the association neocortex. The corticobasal nuclear group of the amygdaloid complex, closely connected with the posterior hippocampal formation, entorhinal cortex and association neocortex, is more usually affected in AD than is the centromedial group, which is less association related (Jamada and Mahraein 1968; Stephan and Andy 1977; Kemper 1984). Regions of the basal forebrain are frequently pathological. The medial septal nucleus, which exchanges fibers with the posterior cingulate gyrus and hippocampal formation, is often affected (Arendt et al. 1985), as is the nucleus basalis of Meynert, which provides most of the cholinergic innervation to the neocortex (Whitehouse et al. 1982; Mesulam et al. 1983; Arendt et al. 1985).

Additionally affected nuclear groups in AD usually are connected with the neocortex. Thus, cortically projecting serotonergic neurons within the dorsal raphe nuclei are affected, as compared with the central superior nucleus (Zweig et al. 1988). Furthermore, dorsally situated noradrenergic neurons within the locus coeruleus (as compared with central neurons which project to the basal ganglia, cerebellum and spinal cord) are lost in the AD brain (Marcyniuk et al. 1986; Mann et al. 1987). The thalamus, caudate nucleus and substantia nigra are less frequently involved. The olfactory bulb, which regresses along the ascending primate scale and has connections with the amygdaloid complex, is also pathological (Mann et al. 1988).

The paired helical filaments of neurofibrillary tangles contain an abnormally phosphorylated, microfilament-associated protein tau, the protein ubiquitin, and high molecular weight protein aggregates (Grundke-Iqbal et al. 1986). These filaments are also found in the neurites of senile plaques. A precursor, a nonphosphorylated tau-like neurofilament protein, has been demonstrated within neurons of layers III and V of the association neocortices, the subiculum, layers II and IV of the entorhinal cortex, and the pyramidal and hilar regions of the hippocampus, all of which demonstrate neurofibrillary tangles in AD (Morrison et al. 1987). When the tangles are evident, however, labeling of the nonphosphorylated precursor disappears.

Alzheimer's disease is accompanied by brain atrophy and neuronal loss. Even early in its clinical course, progressive ventricular dilatation can be demonstrated by serial quantitative computed tomography (Creasey et al. 1986 and this volume; Luxenberg et al., 1987). In the postmortem AD brain, atrophy is more severe in association than in primary cortical regions (Najlerahim and Bowen 1988; Bowen et al.; this volume), where it is evidenced as reduced thickness and reduced length of the cortical ribbon (Duyckaerts et al. 1985; Mann et al. 1985). Neuronal loss in subcortical structures frequently is correlated with plaque, tangle or cell counts in connected cortical areas (Mann et al. 1985; Arendt et al. 1985).

Down's syndrome (trisomy 21) subjects older than 35 years of age display the characteristic neuropathology of AD, although neurofibrillary tangles with paired helical filaments may occur years after high numbers of senile plaques appear in the Down's syndrome brain (Burger and Vogel 1973; Wisnieswki et al. 1985; Mann and Esiri 1989; Schapiro et al. this volume). Furthermore, the topography of neuropathology in the Down's syndrome brain does not differ from the topography in brains of AD patients (Ball and Nuttall 1981; Mann et al. 1984, 1987; Casanova et al. 1985; Schapiro et al., 1986; Marcyniuk et al. 1988). Finally, functional, metabolic and neurochemical disturbances in demented older Down's syndrome subjects are quite similar to those found in AD patients (see below) (Schapiro et al., this volume). These correspondences attest to the similarity of the neurodegenerative processes in Down's syndrome and AD (see "Discussion" below).

Brain Metabolism and Cognition in AD

Positron emission tomography studies of $rCMR_{glc}$ in patients with AD clearly demonstrate early and selective involvement of the association, as compared with primary sensory and motor, cortices in this disorder. In our research program at the Laboratory of Neurosciences, $rCMR_{glc}$ was studied in relation to severity of dementia in AD patients and in age-matched healthy controls. PET was performed on subjects at rest and with reduced visual and auditory inputs, using an ECAT II scanner (ORTEC, Life Sciences, Oak Ridge, TN; FWHM = 17 mm). The AD patients were screened for illnesses other than AD which might contribute to cerebral dysfunction, and the controls were screened very carefully as well. AD (possible or probable) was diagnosed according to NINCDS-ADRDA criteria for choosing patients for research purposes (McKhann et al. 1984). Severity of dementia was assessed with the Mini-Mental State Examination (Folstein et al., 1975); mild, score = 21–30; moderate, score = 11–20; severe, score = 0–10. Subjects were also administered an extensive neuropsychological test battery (Wechsler 1955; Haxby et al. 1986).

Mean scores derived from this battery are summarized in Table 4 for mildly and moderately demented AD patients. Whereas moderately demented patients differed from controls on a wide range of neuropsychological tests, mildly demented patients differed only on the tests of memory ($p < 0.01$). Indeed, a significant and isolated memory impairment, with normal scores on all tests of language and visuospatial function, characterized five of the ten mildly demented patients in Table 4 (Haxby et al. 1986).

Differences between mean $rCMR_{glc}$ values in mildly demented AD patients and controls were difficult to demonstrate statistically because of the large standard deviation of absolute PET data (Duara et al. 1986). However, standard deviations could be reduced to about 5% of the means by calculating ratios of

Table 4. Cognitive test scores in mild and moderate AD[a]

Test	N	Test scores		
		Controls	Mild AD(10)[b]	Moderate AD(12)
Mattis dementia rating scale	16	141 ± 3	131 ± 6	110 ± 18[c,d]
Wechsler memory scale				
Delayed story recall	23	17.6 ± 5.7	2.6 ± 3.7[c]	0.8 ± 1.1[c]
Delayed figure production	23	6.5 ± 3.3	0.8 ± 1.1[c]	0.3 ± 0.8[c]
WAIS				
Full scale IQ	25	125 ± 11	117 ± 8	85 ± 15[c,d]
Verbal comprehension DQ	25	127 ± 11	122 ± 9	96 ± 18[c,d]
Memory and distractibility DQ	15	118 ± 13	114 ± 9	86 ± 14[c,d]
Perceptual organization DQ	25	119 ± 14	108 ± 13	76 ± 19[c,d]
Syntax comprehension (max = 26)	23	24.2 ± 2.5	22.7 ± 2.4	15.8 ± 5.4[c,d]
Boston naming (max = 43)	17	37.6 ± 5.7	35.7 ± 6.5	23.8 ± 9.1[c,d]
Controlled word association	24	40 ± 14	30 ± 8	23 ± 13[e]
Extended range drawing (max = 24)	22	20.6 ± 2.6	18.5 ± 4.1	11.7 ± 4.8[c,d]
Benton facial recognition	25	44.6 ± 3.8	43.7 ± 3.2	40.3 ± 5.4[e]

[a] Data from Haxby et al. (1986)
[b] Number of subjects in parentheses; DQ, factor deviation quotient
[c] Mean $\pm$ SD significantly less than control mean: $p < 0.001$
[d] Mean significantly less than in mild AD: $p < 0.001$
[e] Mean $\pm$ SD significantly less than control mean: $p < 0.01$

Table 5. Relative metabolic rates in AD[a]

Metabolic ratio	Control (30)[b]	Mild AD(12)	Moderate AD(15)	Severe AD(8)
Parietal association sensorimotor	0.93 ± 0.05	0.83 ± 0.09[c]	0.85 ± 0.09[c]	0.72 ± 0.08[c]
Frontal association sensorimotor	0.97 ± 0.07	0.94 ± 0.06	0.92 ± 0.11	0.87 ± 0.18[c]
Lateral temporal association occipital	0.85 ± 0.08	0.76 ± 0.11[c]	0.77 ± 0.11[c]	0.66 ± 0.09[c]

[a] Data from Haxby et al. (1986)
[b] Number of subjects in parenthesis
[c] Mean $\pm$ SD differs from control by Bonferroni t test ($p < 0.05$)

metabolic rates of two brain regions. Thus, as illustrated by Table 5, ratios of association to primary $rCMR_{glc}$ values indicated that the parietal and lateral temporal association cortices were metabolically abnormal even in mildly and moderately demented AD patients, and remained functionally disturbed throughout the course of the disease (Haxby et al. 1986; Rapoport et al. 1986). Indeed, even in severely demented AD patients, primary sensory and motor neocortices, and thalamic and basal ganglia regions, were metabolically more active than were the association neocortices (Fig. 1).

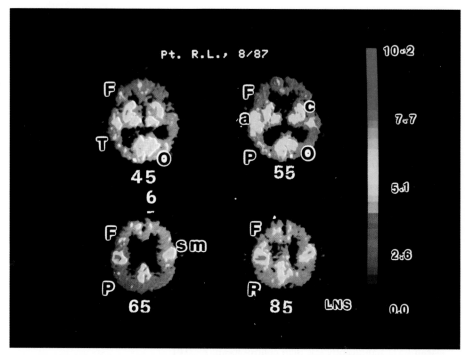

Fig. 1. Position emission tomography scan from severely demented patient with AD. rCMR$_{glc}$, derived with a Scanditronix tomograph (Uppsala, Sweden, FWHM = 6 mm), in units of mg · 100 g^{-1} · min^{-1}. High metabolic rates are retained in the primary sensorimotor cortex (*sm*), primary visual cortex (*o*), primary auditory cortex (*a*) and caudate and lenticular nuclei (*c*), but are reduced elsewhere in the brain. *P*, parietal lobe; *F*, frontal cortex; *T*, temporal cortex; *O*, occipital cortex. (Laboratory of Neurosciences, National Institute on Aging)

Asymmetry of Brain Metabolism and Cognitive Discrepancy in AD

Heterogeneity of metabolic and cognitive deficits characterizes AD patients (Grady et al. 1989 b; Haxby, this volume). Thus, methods in addition to region-by-region comparisons of rCMR$_{glc}$-derived means are needed to identify individual patterns of cognitive and metabolic dysfunction in AD patients and to correlate these patterns, especially early in the course of disease. To do this, Haxby et al. (1985) defined a metabolic asymmetry index (%) for homologous right and left brain regions,

$$\text{Asymmetry index} = \frac{\text{rCMR}_{glc,\,right} - \text{rCMR}_{glc,\,left}}{[\text{rCMR}_{glc,\,right} + \text{rCMR}_{glc,\,left}]/2} \times 100 \tag{1}$$

and correlated metabolic asymmetries in individual patients with discrepancies in relevant cognitive test scores.

Asymmetry indices were calculated for mildly and moderately demented AD patients and for healthy controls, from rCMR$_{glc}$ data obtained with an ECAT II tomograph. Significantly greater variances of asymmetry were demonstrated

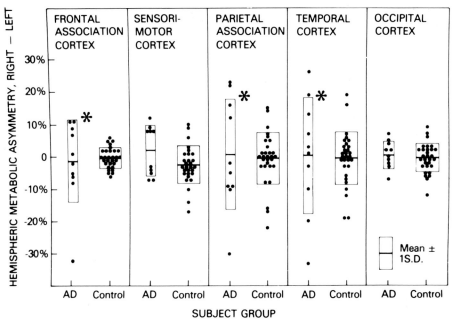

Fig. 2. Metabolic asymmetry (Eq. 1, text) in each of five cortical regions in mildly–moderately demented AD patients and controls. Values are right minus left $rCMR_{glc}$ values, divided by the mean (%). *, coefficient of variation differs from control value. ECAT II data from Haxby et al. (1985)

Table 6. Metabolic asymmetry scores in AD patients[a]

Glucose utilization asymmetry index	Control (29)[b]	Mild AD (10)	Moderate AD (12)
Frontal association cortex	0.00 ± 0.03	-0.01 ± 0.08[c]	-0.02 ± 0.12[c]
Parietal association cortex	0.00 ± 0.06	0.00 ± 0.12[e]	0.02 ± 0.14[c]
Lateral temporal association cortex	-0.01 ± 0.08	-0.05 ± 0.18[d]	-0.04 ± 0.19[c]

[a] Data from Haxby et al. (1986)
[b] Number of subjects in parenthesis. Mean $\pm$ SD is given
[c] Variance is greater than in controls: $p < 0.001$
[d] Variance is greater than in controls: $p < 0.01$
[e] Variance is greater than in controls: $p < 0.05$

($p < 0.05$, asterisks in figure), as compared with controls, in the frontal, parietal, and temporal association regions, but not in the sensorimotor or occipital cortices (Fig. 2; Haxby et al. 1985), indicating that AD selectively involves the association neocortices while sparing comparatively primary and motor regions. When the AD patients were divided according to dementia severity, both the mildly and moderately demented patients were shown to have increased variance of asymmetry in the association neocortices, as compared with controls (Table 6; Haxby et al., 1986). Thus, the association, but not primary sensory or motor, neocortices are distinctly abnormal very early in the course of AD.

Studies of patients with focal brain damage suggest that syntax comprehension, mental arithmetic and immediate verbal memory are related to left parietal and temporal functions, whereas visuospatial construction is related to right parietal function (Benton 1985; Haxby et al. 1985, 1986). To see whether the metabolic asymmetries in AD corresponded to appropriate neocortically mediated cognitive deficits, Haxby et al. (1986) used the Syntax Comprehension Test to test left neocortical function, and the Extended Range Drawing Test to examine right neocortical function. AD patients were ranked separately on the test scores; the difference between the ranks was calculated as a "syntax/drawing discrepancy."

Consistent with Table 4, which demonstrates significant deficits in neocortically mediated cognitive function in moderately but not in mildly demented AD patients, the metabolic asymmetry index was correlated significantly and appropriately with the syntax/drawing discrepancy index in moderately demented patients, but not in mildly demented patients or controls (Table 7). Correlations were significant for the frontal and parietal association neocortices, but not for the lateral temporal or sensory or motor regions; a lower left-sided $rCMR_{glc}$ corresponded to a worse language score, and a lower right-sided $rCMR_{glc}$ corresponded to a worse visuoconstruction test score.

These cross-sectional results suggest that early metabolic dysfunction in association regions of AD patients precedes and predicts the deficits in language and visuospatial performance that later appear. Subsequent longitudinal studies have confirmed this conclusion (Grady et al. 1986, 1988; Haxby et al., submitted, and this volume). Indeed, in individual AD patients studied repeatedly over extended periods of time, it was shown that: (1) the direction of metabolic asymmetry is constant in a given AD patient, (2) the magnitude of metabolic asymmetry increases with time, and (3) the heterogeneous metabolic asymmetries that appear early in the disease precede and accurately predict the heterogeneous deficits in neocortically mediated functions that later appear and establish the individual dementia profile.

Table 7. Correlations between right-left metabolic asymmetries and drawing/syntax comprehension discrepancy [a]

Cortical region	Controls (N = 30)	Mild AD (N = 12)	Moderate AD (N = 15)
Frontal association	−0.30	−0.01	0.71 [b]
Parietal association	−0.11	−0.20	0.73 [b]
Lateral temporal association	−0.08	0.01	0.49

[a] Data from Haxby et al. (1986) Positive correlation indicates that better drawing capacity is correlated with relatively higher right-sided metabolism
[b] $p < 0.05$

Conclusions

A Phylogenic Hypothesis for AD

Glucose metabolism in the association neocortices is disturbed early and through-out the course of AD. Metabolic asymmetries precede and predict appropriate deficits in neocortically mediated cognitive functions that appear consistently in moderately demented patients. Dysfunction of the association neocortices in life, furthermore, corresponds to the selective distribution of neurofibrillary tangles in the postmortem AD brain and to regional cortical atrophy. The postmortem brain, in addition, displays neuropathology in non-neocortical regions closely related, functionally and anatomically, with the association neocortices. These regions belong mainly to System I (Table 1), which comparative anatomical data suggest underwent integrated phylogeny during evolution of higher primates, particularly of hominids.

This topographic distribution of brain dysfunction during life, and of neu-ropathology postmortem, suggests that AD is a phylogenic neurodegenerative disease of higher primates, possibly only of humans (Rapoport 1988 a, b, 1989). Consequently, it has been argued that vulnerability of the brain to AD was introduced into the primate genome during evolution of higher primates, leading to potential for degeneration of System I and other neocortically related regions. Several pieces of evidence are consistent with this proposal.

Insofar as AD selectively affects the association neocortices and non-neocor-tical regions to which they are connected, the disease should be most evident in higher primates. Indeed, in its full-blown form, it has been demonstrated only in man. Furthermore, neurofibrillary tangles with paired helical filaments are found in large quantities in the AD brain, but are absent from the nonhuman brain. Senile (neuritic) plaques in AD are distinct from those in nonhuman brains in that they contain the characteristic paired helical filaments (Terry and Wisniewski 1972; Selkoe et al. 1987).

Alzheimer's disease could have appeared following an evolutionary change in the primate genome, which is consistent with evidence for genetic factors in its pathogenesis. For example, AD can be familial with autosomal dominant trans-mission (Heston et al. 1981; Bird et al. 1988). Chromosome 21 has been implicat-ed in some cases of early-onset familial AD (although not in other familial cases) (St George-Hyslop et al. 1987; Roses et al. 1988; Schellenberg et al. 1988). AD pathology is observed invariably in older subjects with trisomy 21 (Wiśniewski et al. 1985), suggesting a genetic basis involving chromosome 21 for at least some types of the disease. Brains of Down's syndrome subjects older than 40 years exhibit neurochemical abnormalities, and neuropathology with the same density, chemical and antigenic properties, and regional topography as do brains of AD patients (Ball and Nuttall 1981; Mann et al. 1984; Casanova et al. 1985; Wiś-niewski et al. 1985; Schapiro et al. this volume). In life, glucose metabolism is abnormal in the association, but not sensory or motor, neocortices of older demented Down's syndrome subjects (Schapiro et al. 1986, and this volume).

Regulatory Mutations and Altered Gene Expression

Rapid evolution of the brain in higher primates, involving the process of integrated phylogeny, probably did not arise by point mutations coding for structural proteins, but rather by genomic changes leading to increased or otherwise altered expression of genes coding for products in the association neocortices and their connections (King and Wilson 1975; Wilson 1985; Rapoport 1988 a, b, 1989). These events might have included regulatory mutations, leading to altered expression of a regulatory enzyme, growth or recognition factor within association regions; gene duplication, causing a discontinuous increase in expression of regulatory proteins; or chromosomal rearrangement, changing gene expression by altering gene position within a chromosome. Indeed, although nuclear DNA differs by less than 1% between man and the chimpanzee, multiple gene rearrangements distinguish the genomes of these species (King and Wilson 1975; De Grouchy et al. 1978).

A model which is consistent with the hypothesis that AD is a phylogenic disease and related to an evolutionary change in gene expression has been proposed (Rapoport 1988 a, b, 1989). The likelihood of disease in an individual lifetime is predicted by a genomic character function composed of genes x_j, each multiplied by number n_j in the genome, expression e_j (between 0 and 1) and environmental or other factors, a_j,

$$G(x) = a_1 e_1 n_1 x_1 + a_2 e_2 n_2 x_2 + \ldots a_j e_j n_j x_j \ldots \tag{2}$$

Different alleles, causing protein polymorphism, make the value of $G(x)$ "distributed" within a species. In Down's syndrome, $n_j = 3$ if x_j is homozygous and on the 21q22 region of chromosome 21. A discordance rate of 60% in monozygotic twins, one of whom has AD (Nee et al. 1987), emphasizes the importance of variable expression and environmental factors in $G(x)$.

Figure 3 (bottom) illustrates hypothetical $G(x)$ distributions in the chimpanzee (*Pan*), modern *Homo sapiens* and two nonextant intermediate species. It is assumed that hominid speciation was accompanied by a progressive increase in the species average for $G(x)$. Figure 3 (top) gives the likelihood of getting AD in an individual lifetime, which increases with $G(x)$ above a threshold value (identified by arrows). This likelihood is taken as 0 in *Pan* and, in modern man, 6.4% in the general human population, 19% – 23% and 45% in individuals with family risk (considered to represent 40% of the population), and 100% in Down's syndrome (Heston et al. 1981; Wiśniewski et al. 1985). Selective vulnerability is explained by the fact that $G(x)$ increased pari passu with altered expression of some genes coding for proteins in vulnerable brain association regions, implying that some of the genes which promoted evolution of these regions contribute to the value of $G(x)$.

One of several regulatory mutations may have occurred during higher primate evolution, increasing the value of $G(x)$. For example, a regulatory mutation could have altered the regional expression of surface recognition or adhesion molecules (SAMs or CAMs) (Edelman 1987), or of neurotrophic factors which promoted integrated phylogeny. For example, nerve growth factor influences the integrity of the septal-basal forebrain complex, together with its hippocampal and neocor-

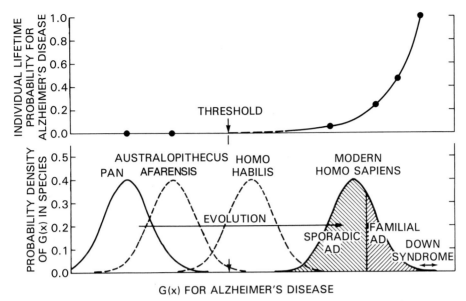

Fig. 3. Genomic character function $G(x)$ for AD, in relation to hominid speciation and likelihood of developing AD in an individual lifetime. *Bottom,* normal distributions for $G(x)$ in different individual species. *Top,* individual likelihood for AD as a function of $G(x)$. *Arrows* indicate threshold value of $G(x)$ above which disease has a finite likelihood. (Rapoport 1989)

tical projection areas (Large et al. 1966; Kromer 1987). Consequently, increased trophic effects of nerve growth factor on basal forebrain neurons may have accelerated phylogeny of these systems in higher primates.

A regulatory mutation could also have promoted brain accumulation of the amyloid precursor protein which contains a protease inhibitor (Palmert et al. 1988; Abraham et al. 1988), as the mRNA for this protein is expressed more in the association than in primary sensory and motor cortices of the human AD brain (Neve et al. 1988 b). The growth-associated protein, GAP-43, is also expressed preferentially in association regions of the human brain (Neve et al. 1988 a). Indeed, levels of mRNA for this neuron-specific phosphoprotein, linked to plasticity of synaptic connections, are high in layer 2 of the association neocortex and in hippocampal pyramidal cells, but low in primary sensory neocortices, several brainstem structures and the caudate putamen. Increased mRNA levels may have resulted from a regulatory mutation of the gene for GAP-43, or of a gene for nerve growth factor or glucocorticoids, both of which can regulate GAP-43 gene expression (Federoff et al. 1988).

A regulatory mutation could have altered the central metabolism of somatostatin 14 or 28 (Davis et al. 1988), or have enhanced accumulation of neurofibrillary tangles with paired helical filaments by increasing phosphorylation of tau, or by reducing dephosphorylation of a phosphorylated derivative (Grundke-Iqbal et al. 1986; Selkoe et al. 1987). In this regard, the gene coding for the S100β protein, which influences tau phosphorylation, has recently been identified on human chromosome 21 (Allore et al. 1988; Baudier and Cole 1988).

References

Abraham CR, Selkoe DJ, Potter H (1988) Immunochemical identification of the serine protease inhibitor alpha 1-antichymotrypsin in the brain amyloid deposits of Alzheimer's disease. Cell 52:487–501

Alexander GE, DeLong MR, Strick PL (1986) Parallel organization of functionally segregated circuits linking basal ganglia and cortex. Ann Rev Neurosci 9:357–381

Allore R, O'Hanlon D, Price R, Neilson K, Willard HF, Cox DR, Marks A, Dunn RJ (1988) Gene encoding the β subunit of S100 protein is on chromosome 21: implications for Down syndrome. Science 239:1311–1313

Andy OJ, Stephan H (1966) Septal nuclei in primate phylogeny. A quantitative investigation. J Comp Neurol 126:157–170

Arendt T, Bigl V, Tennstedt A, Arendt A (1985) Neuronal loss in different parts of the nucleus basalis is related to neuritic plaque formation in cortical target areas in Alzheimer's disease. Neuroscience 14:1–14

Ball MJ, Fisman M, Hachinski V, Blume W, Fox A, Kral VA, Kirshen AJ, Fox H, Merskey H (1985) A new definition of Alzheimer's disease: a hippocampal dementia. Lancet 1:14–16

Ball MJ, Nuttal K (1981) Topography of neurofibrillary tangles and granulovacuoles in hippocampi of patients with Down's syndrome: quantitative comparisons with normal ageing and Alzheimer's disease. Neuropathol Appl Neurobiol 7:13–20

Baudier J, Cole RD (1988) Interactions between the microtubule-associated τ proteins and S100β regulate τ phosphorylation by the Ca^{2+}/calmodulin-dependent protein kinase II. J Biol Chem 263:5876–5883

Baxter LR Jr, Phelps ME, Mazziotta JC, Guze BH, Schwartz JM, Selin CE (1987) Local cerebral glucose metabolic rates in obsessive compulsive disorder. Arch Gen Psychiatry 44:211–218

Benton A (1985) Visuoperceptual, visuospatial and visuoconstructive disorders. In: Heilman KM, Valenstein E (eds) Clinical neuropsychology, 2nd ed. Oxford University Press, Oxford, pp 115–129

Bird TD, Lampe TH, Nemens EJ, Miner GW, Sumi SM, Schellenberg GD (1988) Familial Alzheimer's disease in American descendants of the Volga Germans: probable genetic founder effect. Ann Neurol 23:25–31

Brun A, Gustafson L (1976) Distribution of cerebral degeneration in Alzheimer's disease. A clinico-pathological study. Arch Psychiatr Nervenkr 223:15–33

Burger PC, Vogel FS (1973) The development of pathologic changes of Alzheimer's disease and senile dementia in patients with Down's syndrome. Am J Pathol 73:457–476

Casanova MF, Walker LC, Whitehouse PJ, Price DL (1985) Abnormalities of the nucleus basalis in Down's syndrome. Ann Neurol 18:310–319

Creasey H, Schwartz M, Frederickson H, Haxby JV, Rapoport SI (1986) Quantitative computed tomography in dementia of the Alzheimer type. Neurology 36:1563–1568

Darwin C (1871) The descent of man. In: Hutchins RM (ed) Great books of the western world. Darwin. William Benton, Chicago, 49:pp 1–659

Davis TP, Davies P, Culling-Berglund AJ, Malek E, Gillespie T (1988) Central metabolism of somatostatin 14 and 28 is altered in Alzheimer's disease. Abstr Soc Neurosci 14:155

De Grouchy J, Turleau C, Finaz C (1978) Chromosomal phylogeny of the primates. Annual Rev Genet 12:289–328

Duara R, Grady CL, Haxby JV, Sundaram M, Cutler NR, Heston L, Moore A, Schlageter NL, Larson S, Rapoport SI (1986) Positron emission tomography in Alzheimer's disease. Neurology 36:879–887

Duyckaerts C, Hauw J-J, Piette F, Rainsard C, Poulain V, Berthaux P, Escourolle R (1985) Cortical atrophy in senile dementia of the Alzheimer type is mainly due to a decrease in cortical length. Acta Neuropathol (Berl) 66:72–74

Edelman GM (1987) Neural darwinism. The theory of neuronal group selection. Basic Books, New York, pp 1–371

Federoff HJ, Grabczyk ED, Fishman MC (1988) Dual regulation of GAP-43 gene expression by nerve growth factor and glucocorticoids. J Biol Chem 263:19290–19295

Folstein MF, Folstein SE, McHugh PR (1975) "Mini-mental state". A practical method for grading the cognitive state of patients for the clinician. J Psychiat Res 12:189–198

Gorry JD (1963) Studies on the comparative anatomy of the ganglion basale of Meynert. Acta Anat 55:51–104

Grady CL, Berg G, Carson RE, Daube-Witherspoon ME, Friedland RP, Rapoport SI (1989a) Quantitative comparison of cerebral glucose metabolic rates from two positron emission tomographs. J Nucl Med 30:1386–1392

Grady CL, Haxby JV, Horwitz B, Sundaram M, Berg G, Schapiro M, Friedland RP, Rapoport SI (1988) A longitudinal study of the early neuropsychological and cerebral metabolic changes in dementia of the Alzheimer type. J Clin Exp Neuropsychol 10:576–596

Grady CL, Haxby J, Schapiro MB, Kumar A, Friedland RP, Rapoport SI (1989b) Heterogeneity in dementia of the Alzheimer type (DAT): subgroups identified from cerebral metabolic patterns using positron emission tomography (PET). Neurol 39 (Suppl 1):167–168

Grady CL, Haxby JV, Schlageter NL, Berg G, Rapoport SI (1986) Stability of metabolic and neuropsychological asymmetries in dementia of the Alzheimer type. Neurology 36:1390–1392

Grundke-Iqbal I, Iqbal K, Tung Y-C, Quinlan M, Wiśniewski HM, Binder LI (1986) Abnormal phosphorylation of the microtubule-associated protein τ (tau) in Alzheimer cytoskeletal pathology. Proc Natl Acad Sci USA 83:4913–4917

Haxby JV, Duara R, Grady CL, Cutler NR, Rapoport SI (1985) Relations between neuropsychological and cerebral metabolic asymmetries in early Alzheimer's disease. J Cereb Blood Flow Metab 5:193–200

Haxby JV, Grady CL, Duara R, Schlageter N, Berg G, Rapoport SI (1986) Neocortical metabolic abnormalities precede non-memory cognitive deficits in early Alzheimer's-type dementia. Arch Neurol 43:882–885

Heindel WC, Salmon DP, Shults CW, Walicke PA, Butters N (1989) Neuropsychological evidence of multiple implicit memory systems: a comparison of Alzheimer's, Huntington's, and Parkinson's disease patients. J Neurosci 9:582–587

Heston LL, Mastri AR, Anderson VE, White J (1981) Dementia of the Alzheimer type. Clinical genetics, natural history, and associated conditions. Arch Gen Psychiat 38:1085–1090

Horwitz B, Grady CL, Schlageter NL, Duara R, Rapoport SI (1987) Intercorrelations of regional cerebral glucose metabolic rates in Alzheimer's disease. Brain Res 407:294–306

Huang S-C, Phelps ME, Hoffman EJ, Sideris K, Selin CJ, Kuhl DE (1980) Non-invasive determination of local cerebral metabolic rate of glucose in man. Amer J Physiol 238:E69–E82

Hughlings Jackson J (1884) In: Taylor J (ed) Selected writings of John Hughlings Jackson. Evolution and dissolution of the nervous system, 1931, vol 2. Basic Books, New York, pp 2–118

Hyman BT, Van Hoesen GW, Damasio AR, Barnes CL (1984) Alzheimer's disease: cell-specific pathology isolates the hippocampal formation. Science 225:1168–1170

Hyman BT, Van Hoesen GW, Kromer LJ, Damasio AR (1986) Perforant pathway changes and the memory impairment of Alzheimer's disease. Ann Neurol 20:472–481

Jamada M, Mahraein P (1968) Verteilungsmuster der senilen Veränderungen im Gehirn. Arch Psychiatr Nervenkr 211:308–324

Kemper T (1984) Neuroanatomical and neuropathological changes in normal aging and in dementia. In: Albert ML (ed), Clinical neurology of aging. Oxford University Press, Oxford, pp 9–52

King M-C, Wilson AC (1975) Evolution at two levels in humans and chimpanzees. Science 188:107–116

Kromer LF (1987) Nerve growth factor treatment after brain injury prevents neuronal death. Science 235:214–216

Large TH, Bodary SC, Clegg DO, Weskamp G, Otten U, Reichardt LF (1986) Nerve growth factor expression in the developing rat brain. Science 234:352–355

Lewis DA, Campbell MJ, Terry RD, Morrison JH (1987) Laminar and regional distributions of neurofibrillary tangles and neuritic plaques in Alzheimer's disease: a quantitative study of visual and auditory cortices. J Neurosci 7:1799–1808

Luria AR (1973) The working brain. An introduction to neuropsychology. Basic Books, New York, pp 1–398

Luxenberg JS, Haxby JV, Creasey H, Sundaram M, Rapoport SI (1987) Rate of ventricular enlargement in dementia of the Alzheimer type correlates with rate of neuropsychological deterioration. Neurology 37:1135–1140

Luxenberg JS, Swedo SE, Flament MF, Rapoport J, Friedland RP, Rapoport SI (1988) Neuroanatomic abnormalities in obsessive-compulsive disorder detected with quantitative X-ray computed tomography. Am J Psychiatry 145:1089–1093

Mann DMA, Esiri MM (1989) The pattern of acquisition of plaques and tangles in the brains of patients under 50 years of age with Down's syndrome. J Neurol Sci 89:169–179

Mann DMA, Tucker CM, Yates PO (1988) Alzheimer's disease: an olfactory connection. Mech Ageing Develop 42:1–15

Mann DMA, Yates PO, Marcyniuk B (1984) Alzheimer's presenile dementia, senile dementia of Alzheimer type and Down's syndrome in middle age form an age related continuum of pathological changes. Neuropathol Appl Neurobiol 10:185–207

Mann DMA, Yates PO, Marcyniuk B (1985) Correlation between senile plaque and neurofibrillary tangle counts in cerebral cortex and neuronal counts in cortex and subcortical structures. Neurosci Lett 56:51–55

Mann DM, Yates PO, Marcyniuk B (1987) Dopaminergic neurotransmitter systems in Alzheimer's disease and in Down syndrome at middle age. J Neurol Neurosurg Psychiatry 50:341–344

Marcyniuk B, Mann DMA, Yates PO (1986) Loss of nerve cells from locus coeruleus in Alzheimer's disease is topographically arranged. Neursci Lett 64:247–252

Marcyniuk B, Mann DMA, Yates PO, Ravindra CR (1988) Topography of nerve cell loss from the locus coeruleus in middle aged persons with Down's syndrome. J Neurol Sci 83:15–24

McKhann G, Drachman D, Folstein M, Katzman R, Price D, Stadlan EM (1984) Clinical diagnosis of Alzheimer's disease: report of the NINCDS-ADRDA Work Group under the auspices of Department of Health and Human Services Task Force on Alzheimer's disease. Neurology 34:939–944

Mesulam M-M, Mufson EJ, Levey AI, Wainer BH (1983) Cholinergic innervation of cortex by the basal forebrain: cytochemistry and cortical connections of the septal area, diagonal band nuclei, nucleus basalis (substantia innominata), and hypothalamus in the rhesus monkey. J Comp Neurol 214:170–197

Morrison JH, Lewis DA, Campbell MJ, Huntley GW, Benson DL, Bouras C (1987) A monoclonal antibody to non-phosphorylated neurofilament protein marks the vulnerable cortical neurons in Alzheimer's disease. Brain Res 416:331–336

Najlerahim A, Bowen DM (1988) Regional weight loss of the cerebral cortex and some subcortical nuclei in senile dementia of the Alzheimer type. Acta Neuropathol (Berl) 75:509–512

Nee LE, Eldridge R, Sunderland T, Thomas CB, Katz D, Thompson KE, Weingartner H, Weiss H, Julian C, Cohen R (1987) Dementia of the Alzheimer type: clinical and family study of 22 twin pairs. Neurology 37:359–363

Neve RL, Finch EA, Bird ED, Benowitz LI (1988a) Growth-associated protein GAP-43 is expressed selectively in associative regions of the adult human brain. Proc Natl Acad Sci USA 85:3638–3642

Neve RL, Finch EA, Dawes LR (1988b) Expression of the Alzheimer amyloid precursor gene transcripts in the human brain. Neuron 1:669–677

Palmert MR, Golde TE, Cohen ML, Kovacs DM, Tanzi RE, Gusella JF, Usiak MF, Younkin LH, Younkin SG (1988) Amyloid protein precursor messenger RNAs: differential expression in Alzheimer's disease. Science 241:1080–1084

Pearson RCA, Esiri MM, Hiorns RW, Wilcock GK, Powell TPS (1985) Anatomical correlates of the distribution of the pathological changes in the neocortex in Alzheimer disease. Proc Natl Acad Sci USA 82:4531–4534

Rapoport SI (1988a) Brain evolution and Alzheimer's disease. Rev Neurologique (Paris) 144:79–90

Rapoport SI (1988b) A phylogenic hypothesis for Alzheimer's disease. In: Sinet PM, Lamour Y, Christen Y (eds) Genetics and Alzheimer's disease. Springer, Berlin Heidelberg New York, pp 62–88

Rapoport SI (1989) Hypothesis: Alzheimer's disease is a phylogenic disease. Med Hypotheses 29:147–150

Rapoport SI, Horwitz B, Haxby JV, Grady CL (1986) Alzheimer's disease: metabolic uncoupling of associative brain regions. Can J Neurol Sci 13:540–545

Rogers J, Morrison JH (1985) Quantitative morphology and regional and laminar distributions of senile plaques in Alzheimer's disease. J Neurosci 5:2801–2808

Roofe PG, Matzke HA (1968) Introduction to the study of evolution: its relationship to neuropathology. In: Minkler J (ed) Pathology of the nervous system, vol 1. Blakiston, New York, pp 14–22

Roses AD, Pericak-Vance MA, Haynes CS, Haines JL, Gaskell PA, Yamaoka LH, Hung W-Y, Clark CM, Alberts MJ, Lee JE, Siddique T, Heyman AL (1988) Genetic linkage studies in Alzheimer's disease (AD). Neurology 38 (Suppl 1):173

Sarnat HB, Netsky MG (1981) Evolution of the nervous system, 2nd edn. Oxford University Press, Oxford, pp 1–504

Schapiro MB, Haxby JV, Grady CL, Rapoport SI (1986) Cerebral glucose utilization, quantitative tomography, and cognitive function in adult Down syndrome. In: Epstein CJ (ed) The neurobiology of Down syndrome. Raven Press, New York, pp 89–108

Schellenberg GD, Bird TD, Wijsman EM, Moore DK, Boenhnke M, Bryant EM, Lampe TH, Nochlin D, Sumi SM, Deeb SS, Beyreuther K, Martin GM (1988) Absence of linkage of chromosome 21q21 markers to familial Alzheimer's disease. Science 241:1507–1510

Selkoe DJ, Bell DS, Podlisny MB, Price DL, Cork LC (1987) Conservation of brain amyloid proteins in aged mammals and humans with Alzheimer's disease. Science 235:873–877

Stephan H, Andy OJ (1970) The allocortex in primates. In: Noback CR, Montagna W (eds) The primate brain. Adv primatology, vol 1. Appleton-Century-Crofts, New York, pp 109–135

Stephan H, Andy OJ (1977) Quantitative comparison of the amygdala in insectivores and primates. Acta Anat 98:130–153

Stephan H, Bauchot R, Andy OJ (1970) Data on the size of the brain and of various brain parts in insectivores and primates. In: Noback CR, Montagna W (eds) The primate brain. Adv Primatology, Vol 1. Appleton Century Crofts, New York, pp 289–297

Stephan H, Frahm HD, Baron G (1987) Comparison of brain structure volumes in insectivora and primates. VII. Amygdaloid components. J Hirnforsch 28:571–584

St George-Hyslop PH, Tanzi RE, Polinsky RJ, Haines JL, Nee L, Watkins PC, Myers RH, Feldman RG, Pollen D, Drachman D, Growdon J, Bruni A, Foncin J-F, Salmon D, Frommelt P, Amaducci L, Sorbi S, Piacentini S, Stewart GD, Hobbs WJ, Conneally PM, Gusella JF (1987) The genetic defect causing familial Alzheimer's disease maps on chromosome 21. Science 235:885–890

Swedo SE, Schapiro MB, Grady CL, Cheslow DL, Leonard HL, Kumar A, Friedland R, Rapoport SI, Rapoport JL (1989) Cerebral glucose metabolism in childhood-onset obsessive compulsive disorder. Arch Gen Psychiatry 46:518–523

Terry RD, Wiśniewski HM (1972) Ultrastructure of senile dementia and of experimental analogs. In: Gaitz CM (ed) Aging and the brain. Adv behavioral biol, vol 3. Plenum, New York, pp 89–116

Wechsler D (1955) Wechsler adult intelligence scale. Psychological Corporation, New York, pp 1–300

Whitehouse PJ, Price DL, Struble RG, Clark AW, Coyle JT, Delong MR (1982) Alzheimer's disease and senile dementia: loss of neurons in the basal forebrain. Science 215:1237–1239

Wilson AC (1985) The molecular basis of evolution. Sci Am 253:164–173

Wise SP, Jones EP (1977) Cells of origin and terminal distribution of descending projections of the rat somatic sensory cortex. J Comp Neurol 175:129–158

Wise SP, Rapoport JL (1988) Obsessive-compulsive disorder: is it a basal ganglia dysfunction? In: Rapoport JL (ed) Obsessive compulsive disorder in children and adolescents. American Psychiatric Press, Washington DC, pp 327–344

Wiśniewski KE, Wiśniewski HM, Wen GY (1985) Occurrence of neuropathological changes and dementia of Alzheimer's disease in Down's syndrome. Ann Neurol 17:278–282

Zweig RM, Ross CA, Hedreen JC, Steele C, Cadillo JE, Whitehouse PJ, Folstein MF, Price DL (1988) The neuropathology of aminergic nuclei in Alzheimer's disease. Ann Neurol 24:233–242

Cellular Pathology in Alzheimer's Disease: Implications for Corticocortical Disconnection and Differential Vulnerability

J.H. Morrison, P.R. Hof, M.J. Campbell, A.D. De Lima, T. Voigt, C. Bouras, K. Cox, and W.G. Young

Summary

Detailed regional and laminar analyses of the neuropathological lesions in Alzheimer's disease have led several investigators to hypothesize that key corticocortical and hippocampal circuits are compromised. In fact it has been suggested that a global corticocortical disconnection occurs in Alzheimer's disease, thereby disrupting cohesive, integrated cortical functions and leading to dementia. Our efforts in Alzheimer's disease research are proceeding along two related pathways. First, we are analyzing the pathological human cortex to develop a more detailed profile of the morphology and biochemical phenotype of the subset of neocortical neurons that are vulnerable top degeneration and/or neurofibrillary tangle formation. The second research strategy is to use experimental methods in a nonhuman primate to characterize the morphology, biochemical phenotype, and afferents to the pyramidal cells that furnish long corticocortical projections. Our intention is to correlate the results from the monkey experimental analyses with our neuropathological results to further characterize the degree to which the vulnerable corticocortical neurons in Alzheimer's disease represent the human homologue of the corticocortically projecting neurons under study in the monkey. Within this context we have demonstrated that SMI-32, a monoclonal antibody to nonphosphorylated neurofilament protein, labels a subpopulation of pyramidal cells in layers III and V of neocortical association areas. The morphology and location of these neurons suggest that they furnish long corticocortical projections. In addition, combined immunohistochemistry transport studies in monkey demonstrated that certain corticocortically projecting neurons are SMI-32-immunoreactive. The relative proportion of the corticocortical input to a given location that is SMI-32-immunoreactive varies systematically depending on the source of the projection, but up to 85% of the cells furnishing the projection from inferior temporal to dorsal prefrontal cortex are SMI-32-immunoreactive. Combined intracellular injection-retrograde transport studies demonstrated that, while this projection from inferior temporal cortex to dorsal prefrontal cortex may reflect a huge degree of biochemical homogeneity regarding SMI-32, the cells of origin are a morphologically diverse group. Antisera to calcium-binding proteins demonstrated that, while certain pyramidal cells might have heightened vulnerability in Alzheimer's disease, the GABAergic interneurons labeled by antisera to calcium-binding proteins do not display any cell loss in Alzheimer's disease. Thus, the biochemical and anatomical profiles of the vulnerable and pathology-resistant cells in Alzheimer's disease are becoming increasingly comprehensive; however, a precise biochemical or morphological "signature" for vulnerability has not yet emerged.

Introduction

In both structural and functional terms, Alzheimer's disease (AD) is a disease of the cerebral cortex. Structurally, the hallmarks of AD [neuritic plaques (NP), neurofibrillary tangles (NFT), and neuronal degeneration] are most prevalent in cortex or certain nuclei that project heavily to cortex. The neurological deficits seen in AD are in functions such as memory, learning, cognition, and language. These capacities are all uniquely well-developed in humans and, in fact, are dependent upon the association regions within prefrontal, temporal, and posterior parietal cortex that have expanded so dramatically in the human cortex. The most consistent and striking pathological changes in AD are found within these same association cortices along with hippocampal and limbic cortices, suggesting that, just as the phylogenetic development of these cortical regions has allowed for the higher level cortical functions, their destruction deprives the AD patient of those intellectual functions that are uniquely well developed in man. Even though nuclei outside of the cerebral cortex such as the nucleus basalis (cholinergic), locus coeruleus (noradrenergic) and dorsal raphe (serotonergic) have received extensive attention in AD research, their involvement in AD is generally considered within the framework of their extensive projections to cerebral cortex (Rossor 1982; Iversen et al. 1983; Rossor et al. 1984; Collerton 1986).

Several reports have implicated the corticocortical projections in AD. The distribution of pathological markers of AD is not random, nor is it ubiquitous (Kemper 1984). In recent years, several quantitative analyses of NP and NFT distribution in neocortex (Pearson et al. 1985; Rogers and Morrison 1985; Duyckaerts et al. 1986; Lewis et al. 1987; Braak et al. 1989; Hof et al. 1989; Hof et al. in press) and hippocampus (Wilcock and Esiri 1982; Hyman et al. 1986) have stressed the correlations between NP and NFT distribution and the cells of origin of long corticocortical or key hippocampal projections. Based on these data, it has been proposed that a global corticocortical disconnection occurs in AD, leading to a neocortical isolation syndrome that is manifested as dementia (Rogers and Morrison 1985; Morrison et al. 1986; Lewis et al. 1987; Morrison et al. 1987). Further evidence for the heightened vulnerability of long corticocortical projections and high level association cortices has emerged from metabolic studies using positron emission tomography (Rapoport 1987). On a cellular level it has been demonstrated that significant neuronal loss occurs in AD (Terry et al. 1981; Montjoy et al. 1983; Hansen et al. 1988) and that the neuronal loss primarily involves pyramidal cells (Hansen et al. 1988). Furthermore, NFT formation may only occur in pyramidal cells in the neocortex (Braak and Braak 1986), although there is evidence for the involvement of certain nonpyramidal cells as well (Roberts et al. 1985).

Our recent efforts have centered on the cellular pathology of neocortex in AD and the attempt to determine the aspects of the anatomical and biochemical profiles of the pyramidal cells furnishing long corticocortical projections that are crucially linked to their hightened vulnerability in AD. This approach involves both quantitative neuropathological analysis of human cortex and the experimental analysis of corticocortical circuits in nonhuman primate cortex. In addition, the approach is multidimensional in that relevant biochemical, cellular, and anatomical data are considered within the context of cortical circuitry and primate brain organization, with the goal being a detailed, comprehensive analysis of the neurons providing corticocortical projections and their crucial role in AD and the generation of dementia.

Additional Evidence for Involvement of Corticocortical Projections in AD

We hypothesized that if NP and NFT formation represented the disruption of specific corticocortical circuits, and if this disruption represented the major anatomical substrate for the functional deficits seen in AD, then cases should exist where the disconnection as reflected by the distribution of NP and NFT would correlate directly with specific, identifiable neurological deficits. To test this hypothesis, we compard the distribution of NP and NFT in several cases of AD as it normally presents to several rare cases where a visual defect referred to as Balint's syndrome is superimposed on the dementia and memory defects typically seen in AD (Hof et al. 1989; Hof et al., in press). Our hypothesis predicted that the pathology would directly reflect the neurological symptoms, in that the cases with Balint's syndrome would have far more extensive pathology in the visual areas than is generally seen in AD. Pathological analyses have demonstrated that Balint's syndrome generally involves bilateral parieto-occipital lesions caused by infarctions, although our AD cases with Balint's syndrome (ADB) had no evidence of infarction in the parietal or occipital lobe. The clinical symptomatology of this syndrome has been recently reviewed (Hausser et al. 1980) and can be characterized as having three key qualitites: (1) impairment of target pointing under visual guidance (optic ataxia), (2) inability to shift gaze at will toward new visual stimuli (ocular apraxia), and (3) perception and recognition of only parts of the visual field (simultanagnosia). Therefore, the visual deficits in Balint's syndrome involve visuospatial skills and detection of movement rather than form analysis and, as such, involve the occipitoparietal visual pathway, rather than the occipito-inferior temporal pathway (Mishkin et al. 1983; DeYoe and Van Essen 1988). Not only do patients with ADB have a dramatic increase in the number of NFT and NP in occipital visual areas, but also an increase in NP area/mm^2 of tissue section in inferior parietal lobe and a decrease in NFT in prefrontal cortex as compared to normal AD cases (Fig. 1). Neurofibrillary tangle density in area 17 increases from 2.66 ± 0.18 in the superficial layers and 0.66 ± 0.19 in the deep layers of the AD cases of 81.5 ± 17.66 (layers I–IVB) and 58.5 ± 11.44 (IVC–VI)

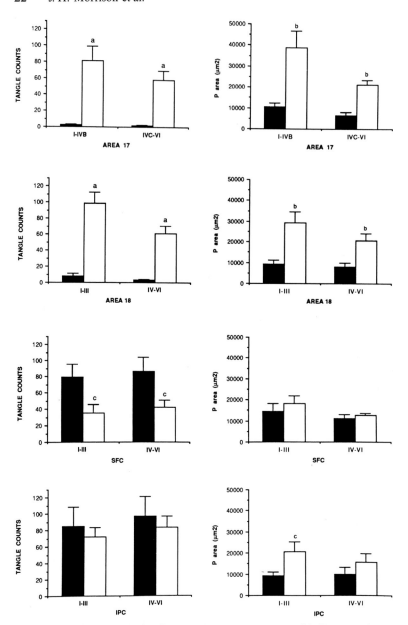

Fig. 1. Quantitative analysis of AD and ADB cases. Neurofibrillary tangle counts/mm^2 (*left column*) and neuritic plaque area (NP, $\mu m^2/mm^2$ of tissue section; *right column*) in superficial and deep layers of area 17, area 18, superior frontal (*SFC*) and inferior parietal (*IPC*) cortices. *Black bars* represent six AD cases, and *white bars* six ADB cases. Results are means ± SEM. *a*, $p < 0.001$; *b*, $p < 0.025$; *c*, $p < 0.01$, two-sided Mann-Whitney U test. (Hof et al. 1989)

in the ADB cases. A similar dramatic increase in NFT density of the ADB cases is seen in both superficial and deep layers of area 18 (7.66±3.33 and 3.16±0.98 to 98.83±13.85 and 61.16±9.19, respectively). In contrast to the dramatic increase in NFT density seen in the occipital areas of the ADB cases, the NFT density is decreased in the superior frontal gyrus (area 9) of the ADB cases as compared to the AD cases (ADB: layers I–III, 35.66±9.68; layers IV–VI, 42.50±8.47. AD: layers I–III, 79.66±16.23; layers IV–VI, 86.50±17.44, Fig. 1). Neurofibrillary tangle counts in the inferior parietal lobe (area 7b) are equivalent in the AD and ADB cases. Neuritic plaque area also is much higher (2.5- to 4-fold) in the superficial and deep layers of 17 and 18 in the ADB cases than in the AD cases, whereas total NP area in the superior frontal gyrus (area 9) is equivalent in the two groups of patients. Total NP area in the inferior parietal lobe (area 7b) is significantly higher in layers I–III of the ADB cases (AD, 9217.12±1941.97; ADB, 20652.00±4746.39, Fig. 1), but is not significantly different in the deep layers. Neuritic plaques counts were also higher in areas 17, 18, and 7b in the ADB brains as compared to AD cases. We have now added additional cases and several frontal and temporal regions to this study, and the findings described above have held up without exception (Hof et al., in press).

Thus, not only has a caudal shift in the distribution of pathological markers occurred, but the increased lesion counts in inferior parietal lobe as well as in the primary and secondary visual cortices suggest that the occipitoparietal stream of connections that subserves visuospatial analysis has been more dramatically disconnected in these cases than is generally the case in AD. These results suggest that multiple subtypes of AD exist. Further, they support the hypothesis that NP and NFT formation involve the loss of specific corticocortical projections and that this loss causes specific functional deficits.

Immunohistochemical Studies with SMI-32

Distribution of SMI-32-Immunoreactive Neurons in Monkey and Normal Human Cortex. SMI-32, a Sternberger-Meyer monoclonal antibody (Sternberger and Sternberger 1983), has been shown to recognize nonphosphorylated epitope on human medium and heavy neurofilament protein subunits (Lee et al. 1988). As a number of monoclonal antibodies to neurofilament proteins have been shown to exhibit cross-reactivity with microtubule-associated proteins, it is significant that this antibody has been shown to lack cross-reactivity to human microtubule-associated proteins (Lee et al. 1988). In an attempt to begin to characterize both the morphology and biochemical phenotype of the vulnerable cortical neurons in AD, we have used SMI-32 for detailed immunohistochemical studies of both monkey and human neocortex and hippocampus. There were two major reasons for choosing this antibody as a probe for the vulnerable cells. First, in preliminary studies this antibody appeared to be a superb marker for pyramidal cells, in monkey and human cortex, and it was clear that the primarily vulnerable cell class was since a discrete subset of pyramidal cells (Morrison et al. 1987; Fig. 2). Second, neurofilament as well as several other cytoskeletal proteins have been

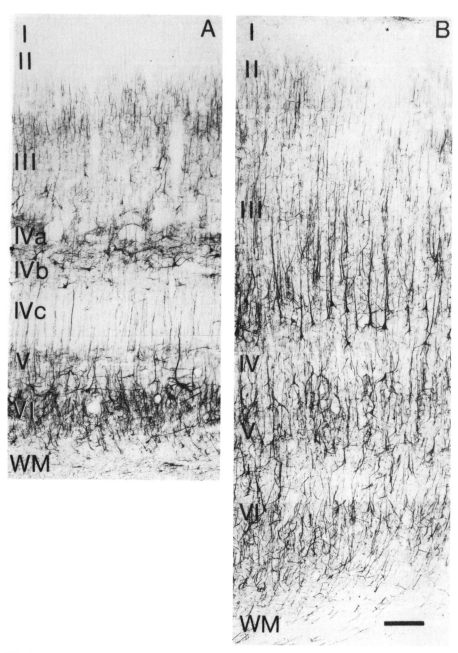

Fig. 2 A, B. Distribution of SMI32-ir neurons in the human primary visual cortex (**A**) and in a visual association area, the posterior inferior temporal cortex (**B**). Note the presence of Meynert cells in layer VI and intensely labeled neurons in layer IVB of the primary visual cortex, and the higher density of SMI32-ir neurons in layers III and V in inferior temporal cortex. *Calibration bar,* 200 μm. (Campbell and Morrison 1989)

implicated in NFT formation; thus, cells with a high content of nonphosphorylated neurofilament protein might be prone to NFT formation.

As expected, SMI-32 immunoreactivity in the primate neocortex was primarily limited to the perikaryon and dendrites of neurons exhibiting a pyramidal cell morphology. However, it was also clear that only a subpopulation of pyramidal neurons was SMI-32-immunoreactive (SMI32-ir; Fig. 2). In addition, there were substantial differences in the intensity of SMI-32 immunoreactivity which were related to cell size: the greater the cell size, the greater the intensity of immunoreactivity (Figs. 3, 4). This relationship was not only evident in the cell body but also was a feature of dendritic immunoreactivity. Quantitative analyses with a confocal microscope demonstrated that this correlation is not an artifact of cell size but, in fact, suggests that the intracellular concentration of neurofilament protein is higher in the larger neurons (Figs. 3, 4; Campbell and Morrison 1989).

We have completed a detailed description of the cellular, laminar and regional characteristics of SMI32-ir cells in certain temporal and occipital areas of both monkey and human cortex (Campbell and Morrison 1989) as well as cingulate and prefrontal cortex. Extensive regional heterogeneity exists in the size, density and laminar distribution of SMI32-ir cells. The distribution patterns match those that have been demonstrated for certain efferent systems. In many cases, the distribution of SMI32-ir cells matched the distribution of corticocortically projecting cells, as demonstrated in transport studies in monkey cortex. For example, in anterior cingulate cortex the labeled cells were restricted to layer V. It has been demonstrated that most long corticocortical projections from anterior cingulate originate in layer V as well (Barbas 1986). Area 9 in the prefrontal cortex, as well as superior and inferior temporal gyri, had a high density of labeled cells in III and V, and corticocortical projections emanate from III and V in these regions (Barbas 1986). The correlation between origins of long corticocortical projections and SMI32-ir neurons was particularly striking in primary visual cortex of both monkey and human. In both species, the large, heavily immunoreactive neurons were restricted to layer IVB and to the Meynert cell class of layer VI, both known to be the site of origin of the projection from area V1 to MT (Van Essen 1985; Shipp and Zeki 1989a). The most important differences across species were that the SMI32-ir cells were larger and more numerous in human than monkey.

Neuropathological Studies with SMI-32

Correlation of SMI32-ir Neurons with Pathological Profiles in AD. The regional and laminar distribution of SMI32-ir neurons suggested that they might represent a significant portion of the cells of origin of long corticocortical projections (Campbell and Morrison 1989).

In addition, in an initial study of the effects of AD on SMI32-ir neurons, we observed that large, intensely SMI32-ir neurons in certain neocortical and hippocampal areas appeared to be highly prone to cell death and/or NFT formation in AD (Morrison et al. 1987; Hof et al. 1988). The laminar distribution of SMI32-ir neurons in visual areas of normal human cortex such as Brodman areas

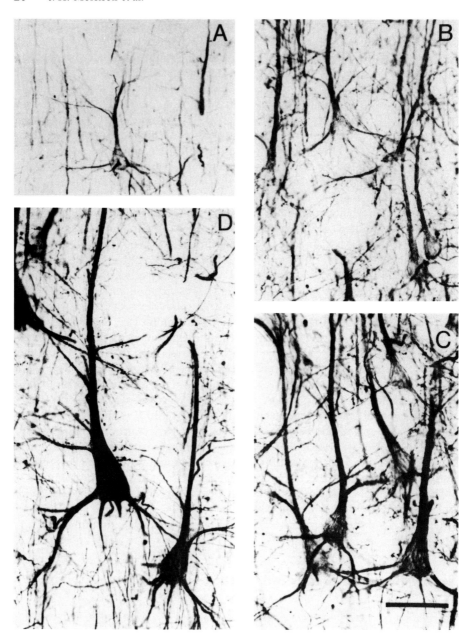

Fig. 3A–D. Photomicrographs from layer III of the human superior temporal cortex showing size-related differences in SMI-32 staining intensity. Note that the intensity of immunoreactivity parallels the increase in cell size (**A–D**). *Calibration bar*, 40 μm. (Campbell and Morrison 1989)

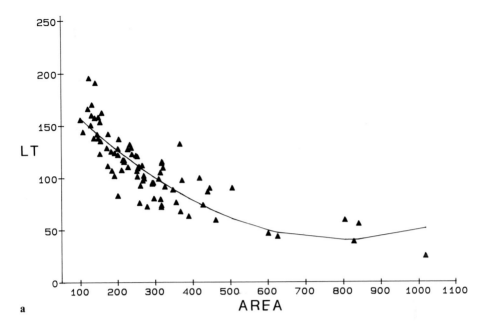

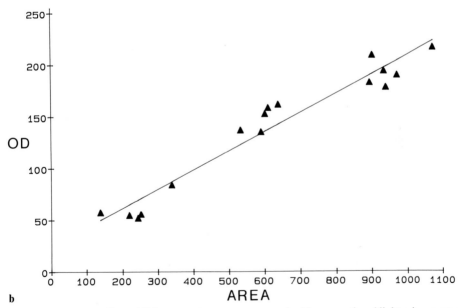

Fig. 4. a Average perikaryal light transmittance as measured with conventional light microscopy (*LT*; $0 =$ black or no transmittance, $255 =$ white or 100% transmittance) versus perikaryal cross-sectional area (μm^2). **b** Average perikaryal optical density as measured with a confocal laser microscope (*OD*; $0 =$ black or no fluorescence, $255 =$ white or maximal fluorescence; 1-μm-thick optical sections) versus perikaryal cross-sectional area (μm^2). The largest labeled cells have a higher OD. Least square-fit analysis, $p < 0.0001$; 81 SMI32-ir cells. Human superior temporal cortex. (Campbell and Morrison 1989)

18 and 20 (V2 and inferior temporal), as well as prefrontal and anterior cingulate cortices, is very similar to the distribution of NFT in these areas. Futhermore, the layers that have high NFT density in an AD brain no longer contain a high density of SMI32-ir neurons. A similar situation exists in parahippocampal areas where layer II of entorhinal cortex and the subiculum have a very high density of SMI32-ir neurons in the healthy human brain, yet are filled with NFT and lack SMI32-ir neurons in an AD brain (Morrison et al. 1987). These observations suggested that SMI32-ir neurons were highly vulnerable in AD, and that they either degenerated in layers and regions with high NFT counts or were prone to NFT formation. These qualitative observations were followed with detailed quantitative studies in which SMI32-ir cell counts were correlated with total cell loss, NFT counts and NP counts.

Quantitative Analysis of SMI32-ir Cell Loss in Superior Frontal and Inferior Temporal Cortices. Detailed quantitative neuropathological studies of SMI32-ir neurons in layers III and V of superior frontal and inferior temporal cortices were conducted on our computer-assisted microscopy system (Hof et al. 1988). These layers and regions were chosen because they have a high density of SMI32-ir neurons in monkey and normal human and are devastated in AD. The following parameters were quantified: (1) SMI32-ir cell counts/mm^2 in layers III and V; (2) SMI32-ir cell size; (3) SMI32-ir cell optical density (for each cell individually); (4) total neuronal counts/mm^2; (5) thickness of layers III and V; (6) NFT counts/ mm^2; and (7) NP counts/mm^2. AD cases were divided into low NFT AD brains (NFT counts less than 30/mm^2) and high NFT AD brains (NFT counts greater than 30/mm^2) and were analyzed as separate groups. In addition, the SMI32-ir neurons were placed in three size categories of perikaryal cross-sectional area: less than 250 mm^2, 250–350 mm^2, and greater than 350 mm^2. The size categorization was done so that we could determine the degree to which vulnerability correlated with cell size.

This quantitative analysis demonstrated that there is an extensive loss of SMI32-ir neurons in layers III and V of both the inferior temporal gyrus and the superior frontal gyrus (Figs. 5, 6). Furthermore the degree of cell loss is related to cell size in that the large neurons are the most affected (up to 90% cell loss; Fig. 6) and the intermediate size class is more susceptible to degeneration than the small size class. Also, the fact that cell loss in the large cell class is equivalent in the low NFT AD and the high NFT AD cases, whereas the small and intermediate size cell classes suffer a further loss in high NFT AD, suggests that the large SMI32-ir cells are particularly vulnerable. The heightened vulnerability of this cell class is further supported by the fact that the average total neuron loss in the low NFT AD cases is 24%, whereas 83% of the large SMI32-ir cells are lost in these cases. Finally, the optical density measurements revealed a highly significant decrease in staining intensity in the remaining SMI32-ir neurons in AD

Fig. 5A–D. SMI32-ir neurons in layers III (A, B) and V (C, D) of the human superior frontal gyrus. A and C are from a control case, whereas panels B and D are from a high NFT AD case. There is a striking cell loss in the AD case. Also, note the difference in SMI32-ir neuron staining intensity in the AD case. *Calibration bar*, 50 μm

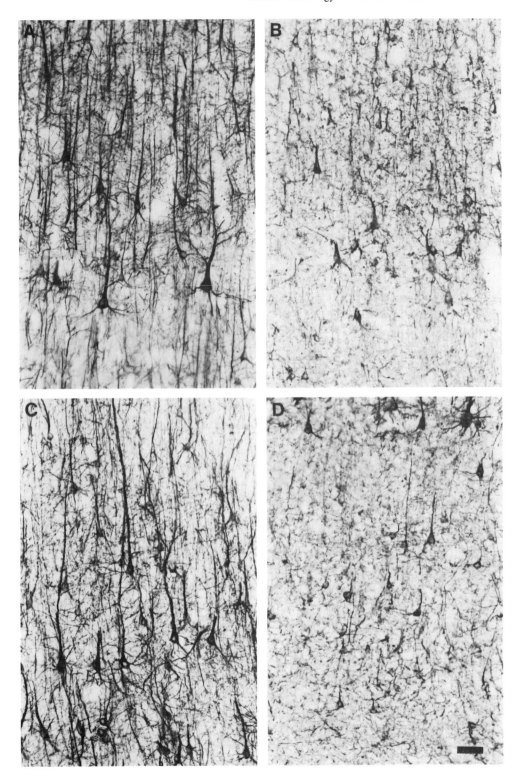

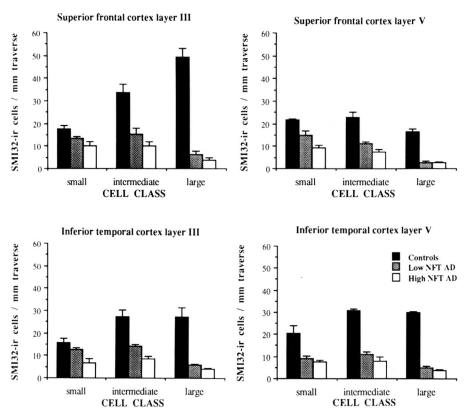

Fig. 6. SMI32-ir neuron counts in layers III and V of human superior frontal and inferior temporal cortices. Results represent means ± SEM from four control, three low NFT AD (less than 30 NFT/mm²), and five high NFT AD (more than 30 NFT/mm²) cases. Size categories: small, < 250 μm²; intermediate, 250–350 μm²; large, > 350 μm². Note that a dramatic cell loss in the large cell class occurs even in the low NFT AD cases ($p < 0.001$) as compared to the intermediate and small cell classes. Statistical significance was between $p < 0.001$ and 0.01, two-sided Mann-Whitney U test

brains as compared to controls, suggesting that either synthesis or phosphorylation of neurofilament protein is disrupted in those cells that remain in AD. Whereas both SMI32-ir cell loss and total neuron loss are strongly correlated with NFT density, neither of these measures of pathology are correlated with NP counts. Although it is likely that some SMI32-ir neurons are prone to NFT formation, we could not determine the relative number of SMI32-ir cells that are lost of NFT formation as opposed to degeneration without NFT.

We have shown in cynomolgus monkey that several long corticocortical projections originate from SMI32-ir neurons, and that the cells of origin of certain projections, such as that from the inferior temporal gyrus to the prefrontal cortex, are 90%–100% SMI32-ir (see below). If the monkey data are considered within the context of the results on SMI32-ir neurons in human cortex presented above, then it appears likely that the human equivalents of the SMI32-ir corticocortically projecting neurons inthe monkey are lost in AD. The biochemical profile of the neurons that are vulnerable in AD needs to be developed, but it appears to include high levels of nonphosphorylated neurofilament proteins in both the soma and dendrites. Neurofilament proteins and other cytoskeletal proteins have been implicated in NFT formation (Perry et al. 1985; Grundke-Iqbal et al. 1986; Joachim et al. 1987; Selkoe 1989). Future studies will be aimed at developing a more comprehensive cytoskeletal profile of the SMI32-ir neurons, as well as pyramidal cells that are not SMI32-ir. Pre- and postsynaptic markers for these neurons must also be identified. Data exist suggesting that the neurotransmitter for corticocortically projecting neurons is glutamate (Conti et al. 1988). Given the demonstrated deficit in glutamate markers in AD (Greenamyre et al. 1985; Hyman et al. 1987), further investigations may reveal that the SMI32-ir neurons are also glutamatergic.

Quantitative Analysis of SMI32-ir Neurons in Visual Areas 17 and 18. Visual impairment is not uncommon in AD (Katz and Rimmer 1989), and may be related to dysfunction of higher level visual processing subserved by visual association cortices in temporal and parietal lobes. In fact, several quantitative studies of NP and NFT distribution in AD have shown that, although visual association cortices contain a high density of NP and NFT, primary visual cortex (area 17) contains numerous NP, but very few NFT (Pearson et al. 1985; Rogers and Morrison 1985; Lewis et al. 1987; Braak et al. 1989; Hof et al. 1989; Hof et al., in press). The one demonstrated exception to this pattern is in cases of AD that also presented with Balint's syndrome (see above). In addition, in contrast to frontal, parietal, and temporal areas, the total neuronal counts in area 17 do not differ between AD and control brains (Mountjoy et al. 1983). Also, in contrast to temporal, parietal and frontal regions, the NFT in area 18 are predominantly restricted to layer III (Lewis et al. 1987; Hof et al. 1989; Hof et al, in press).

The data described above demonstrate that, in areas that have a high density of SMI32-ir neurons such as inferior temporal and superior frontal cortices, there is extensive loss of these neurons in AD and that the extent of the loss is correlated with NFT density. Given these results, two reasonable predictions arise regarding the pathology of SMI32-ir neurons in the occipital cortex. First, given that NFT are rare in area 17 and largely confined to layer III in area 18, we predicted that SMI32-ir neuron loss would be minimal in area 17 and primarily localized to layer III of area 18. Second, it is known that the long projection from 17 to MT originates in layer IVB and from the Meynert cells at the layer V–VI border (Van Essen 1985; Shipp and Zeki 1989a). Similarly, the projection from 18 to MT originates in deep layer III (Shipp and Zeki 1989b). In addition, these layers contain the only heavily SMI32-ir neurons present in 17 (Campbell and Morrison 1989). Therefore, if our hypothesis regarding the vulnerability of long corticocortical projection neurons and SMI32-ir neurons is valid, then any SMI32-ir cell loss that does occur in area 17 should be most pronounced in layer IVB and in the Meynert cell class, and in deep layer III in area 18. To test these predictions, the following parameters were measured in areas 17 and 18 of control and AD brains: (1) SMI-32-ir cell number/mm cortical traverse for all laminae and sublaminae; (2) SMI-32-ir neuron size; (3) SMI-32-ir optical density; (4) NFT number/mm cortical traverse in each layer, (5) NP number/mm cortical traverse in each layer, and (6) full cortical thickness.

The distributions of SMI32-ir cells in areas 17 and 18 differ substantially from each other and from the pattern described in inferior temporal and prefrontal cortices (Hof et al. 1988; Campbell and Morrison 1989). In area 17, the large intensely stained SMI32-ir neurons are largely restricted to layer IVB, to the Meynert cells located at the V–VI border, and to occasional cells in layer III (Fig. 2). Smaller, more lightly stained cells are also present in layers III, V, and VI. In contrast, the large, darkly labeled neurons present in area 18 predominate in the deep portion of layer III, with a few in layer V. Inferior temporal and prefrontal cortices have a significantly higher density of heavily labeled cells in deep layer III than area 18 and, in addition, have a much higher density of labeled cells in layers V and VI (Figs. 2, 5–7).

In contrast to the inferior temporal and prefrontal cortices, the SMI32-ir neuron loss in area 17 and 18 was minimal. In area 17, cell loss was confined to layer IVB and to the Meynert cell class, and averaged 25.4% in these layers. In area 18, the SMI32-ir cell loss was restricted to deep layer III and layer VI and averaged 18.3% in these layers (Fig. 7). Thus, the extensive short corticocortical projection from area 17 to area 18 that emanates from layer III (Van Essen 1985) is presumably not affected in AD, since the lightly immunoreactive cells in layers III, V and VI of area 17 were not damaged in the AD cases. In addition, the lightly labeled cells in layers V and VI in area 17 that probably furnish projections to several subcortical sites (Van Essen 1985) do not appear to be affected in AD.

Given the morphology and distribution of the SMI32-ir cells in area 17, it is very likely that the SMI32-ir neurons in layer IVB and the SMI32-ir Meynert cells represent the cells of origin of the projection to MT. In addition, the projection of area V2 to MT originates from the pyramidal cells in deep layer III (Shipp and Zeki 1989 b), precisely the same location as the vast majority of the darkly stained, large SMI32-ir cells in area 18. The only significant cell loss that has been demonstrated in area 17 is in the SMI32-ir cells of IVB and in the Meynert cell class. Thus, although the projection from 17 to 18 may be intact, and the overall cell loss may appear inconsequential in area 17, it appears likely that two important projections involved in visuomotor skills (namely V1 to MT and V2 to MT) are compromised in AD. This interpretation is dependent upon the SMI-32-ir neurons actually furnishing these projections, and transport studies will provide these data for nonhuman primate. Clearly, the cells of origin of the corticocortical projections are heterogeneous in their biochemical phenotype. Further analyses must be done to more definitively link connectivity with biochemical characteristics, and determine the qualities that confer a selective vulnerability on a given subset of neurons in AD. However, these observations on visual cortex allowed us to demonstrate the possible existence of a chemically defined neuronal subpopulation that is highly vulnerable in AD and that can be correlated with a specific corticocortical projection of known function.

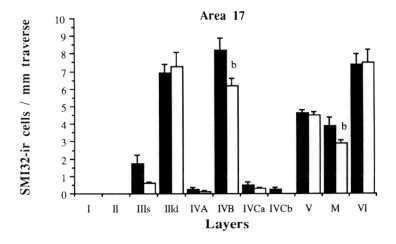

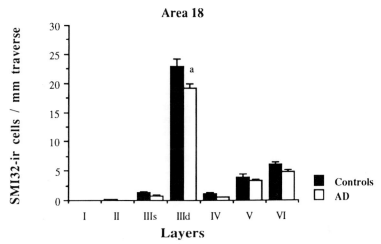

Fig. 7. SMI32-ir neuron counts in area 17 and 18 of the human occipital cortex. Results represent means ± SEM from five control and five AD cases. Note the pathological changes in layer IVB cells and in the Meynert cell class of area 17 and in layer III of area 18. *a*, $p = 0.025$; *b*, $p < 0.05$; *c*, $p = 0.05$, two-sided Mann-Whitney U test

Connectivity Studies

Double-Labeling of Corticocortically Projecting Pyramidal Cells with SMI-32. In previous primate neocortical studies we observed that SMI32-ir pyramidal neurons exhibited a regionally heterogeneous distribution and hypothesized that this resulted from shifts in the representation of SMI32-ir neurons furnishing long corticocortical projections (Campbell and Morrison 1989). We have initiated combined retrograde tracer and immunohistochemical studies in the Macaca fascicularis to test this hypothesis (Campbell et al. 1989). The retrograde tracer

Table 1. Fast blue and double-labeled neuron counts in cortical source regions after tracer injection in the principal sulcus of *Macaca fascicularis*[a]

	Fast blue	Double labeled	%
Ipsilateral principal sulcus			
Layer III	114 ± 21	22 ± 3	18
Layers V–VI	98 ± 15	27 ± 5	27
Contralateral principal sulcus			
Layer III	88 ± 5	23 ± 1	26
Layers V–VI	32 ± 2	10 ± 1	31
Ipsilateral anterior cingulate cortex			
Layer III	1	0	0
Layers V–VI	20 ± 1	10 ± 1	50
Contralateral anterior cingulate cortex			
Layer III	1	0	0
Layers V–VI	14 ± 1	7	50
Ipsilateral intraparietal sulcus			
Layer III	29 ± 3	17 ± 2	58
Layers V–VI	20 ± 2	12 ± 1	60
Ipsilateral superior temporal sulcus			
Layer III	13 ± 2	11 ± 1	85
Layers V–VI	11 ± 1	9 ± 1	82

[a] Fast blue was injected in the principal sulcus of three animals. Results are means $\pm$ SEM from 6 to 15 one-millimeter-wide cortical traverses in each cortical area and represent fast blue only-labeled cell counts and double-labeled (i.e., fast blue plus SMI32-ir) cells counts. The right column represents the percentage of double-labeled neurons. Note the higher proportion of double-labeled cells in areas distant from the injection site, as compared to more local projections

fast blue was injected into the cortical region rostral to the arcuate sulcus and ventral to the principal sulcus, and we determined the number of Fast blue retrogradely labeled neurons and double-labeled neurons (i.e., those containing fast blue and SMI32-ir) and several cortical traverses from each source cortical region (Table 1). These data illustrate: (1) the potential to define distinct subsets of corticocortically projecting neurons based on differences in their molecular constituents, and (2) the degree to which specific corticocortical projections of an area vary in their proportional representation of neuronal subsets so defined. Note that in regions such as the superior temporal sulcus the total number of cells projecting to this field in prefrontal cortex is fewer than from the more local projections, yet the proportion that are SMI32-ir is much higher. In fact, the SMI32-ir double-labeled neurons can be viewed as a subset of the total set of corticocortical projections converging on the injection site. This subset represents a distributed system sharing an important property regarding their biochemical phenotype. Additional transport studies will be needed to further differentiate this subset from the non-SMI32-ir corticocortical projections, further characterize the degree to which they represent a functionally relevant distributed system, and further clarify the rules regarding biochemical and anatomical heterogeneity among corticocortically projecting pyramidal cells.

Intracellular Filling of Corticocortically Projecting Pyramidal Neurons. Cell loading in combination with retrograde transport and chemically specific labeling techniques can be used to determine the biochemical phenotype, morphology and afferents to the corticocortical projection neuron. Such an approach allows for the detailed analysis of the molecular and anatomical profile of a pyramidal cell with a known efferent projection. We have just completed a study in which we have used this technology to characterize the morphology of corticocortically projecting neurons (De Lima et al., in press). This analysis was not carried to the immunohistochemical or ultrastructural level, and therefore does not allow for direct correlation with information on biochemical phenotype. However, we know from the studies outlined above that over 90% of the neurons that furnish the projection analyzed are likely to be SMI32-ir.

We combined intracellular injection of lucifer yellow (LY) in fixed tissue with in vivo retrograde transport of fast blue to study the dendritic morphology of neurons within the inferior temporal gyrus (ITG) that furnish corticocortical projections to the portion of the prefrontal cortex immediately ventral to the principal sulcus (De Lima et al., in press). The fast blue retrogradely labeled cells formed two clearly defined bands within the ITG: a supragranular band that corresponded to layer III, and an infragranular band that corresponded to layers V and VI. After LY intracellular filling, these retrogradely labeled cells projecting to the prefrontal cortex were found to be morphologically very heterogeneous. Although all filled cells had spiny dendrites, they presented a wide range of cell body sizes and dendritic tree morphologies. In layer III, the majority of cells were typical pyramids of various sizes. In layers V–VI, numerous typical pyramidal cells were present. In addition, significant numbers of modified pyramidal forms were found, including vertical and horizontal fusiform cells, asymmetrical pyramids and multipolar cells.

Considering the entire cell population which projects from the ITG to the prefrontal cortex, their dendrites cover the entire cortical depth going from the pial surface to the white matter. As a group, these cells are capable of sampling afferents to all laminar locations. Each individual subgroup, however, covers only a limited portion of the cortical depth and is thus restricted to subsets of afferents. Thus, even when the efferent target is limited to only one of the many ipsilateral cortical targets of the ITG, multiple morphological subtypes contribute to the projection. Furthermore, we know from our other transport studies that virtually all of these neurons are SMI32-ir, even though their morphology may be heterogeneous. Further studies will be directed at determining the afferents to each subtype of corticocortically projecting cell, and the degree to which other cytoskeletal probes reflect the same degree of homogeneity in this population of cells as SMI-32 does.

Thus far, this appears to be an excellent example of the necessity for a multifaceted definition of cell type. As more data of this type accumulate we should be able to construct a system of cell typology in primate cortex that is based on connectivity and biochemical phenotype, as well as location and morphology. In such a scenario a given cell type would be described as not only a cell in a given layer, with certain dendritic and axonal branching patterns, but also in reference to a defined set of connections, and high intracellular levels of certain structural, metabolic or neurotransmitter-related proteins.

Immunohistochemical Studies of Calcium-Binding Proteins

Antibodies to calcium-binding proteins such as parvalbumin are excellent markers for certain nonpyramidal interneurons in monkey and human cortex. Parvalbumin and calbindin both label independent subsets of GABA neurons in neocortex (Hendry et al. 1989). Given the deviation of certain pyramidal cell subtypes

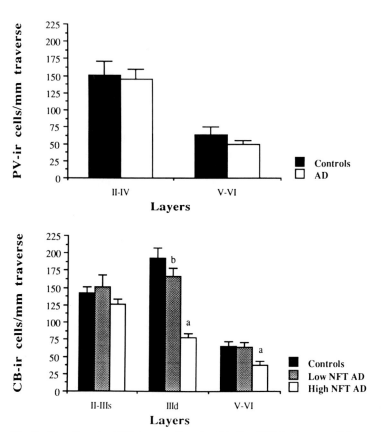

Fig. 8. Parvalbumin- (*PV, top panel*) and calbindin- (*CB, bottom panel*) immunoreactive neuron distribution in human superior frontal cortex. Results represent means ± SEM from four control and eight AD cases (*PV*), and four control, three low NFT AD, and five high NFT AD cases (*CB*). There are no statistically significant differences between control and AD cases for PV-ir neuron counts, whereas there is a striking loss of the CB-ir pyramidal neurons in layer III (*a*, $p < 0.001$; *b*, $p < 0.05$, two-sided Mann-Whitney U test). Note the significant CB-ir cell loss in layers V–VI in the high NFT AD cases. Low and high NFT AD cases as described in Fig. 6

in AD, we investigated the degree to which these nonpyramidal GABAergic neurons are vulnerable as well. Using a monoclonal antibody against the calcium binding protein parvalbumin (Celio et al. 1988), we investigated the possible changes in subpopulation of interneurons in two cortical areas known to be strongly damaged in AD, namely inferior temporal and superior frontal gyri.

No statistically significant differences in the distribution of parvalbumin-immunoreactive (PV-ir) profiles were observed in AD brains as compared to control cases (Morrison et al. 1988). Cellular densities calculated in layers II–IV were similar in AD and control cases in both areas (Fig. 8). There were no differences in PV-ir neuron size between the two brain groups. Very similar values were obtained in layers II–IV and in the prefrontal cortex. These results suggest that PV-ir cells represent a neuronal subset resistant to degeneration, and further support the hypothesis that the pathological process in AD involves specific neuronal subtypes with particular morphological and molecular profiles.

Using a monoclonal antibody to the calcium binding protein calbindin (Celio et al. 1986), we observed in the human prefrontal cortex distinct populations of labeled cells. First, a subset of heavily stained interneurons was located in layers II and superficial III, and in layers V–VI. Second, a subpopulation of pyramidal neurons in the mid and deep parts of layer III displayed a less intense, punctate staining pattern. A quantitative analysis demonstrated that the interneurons in the superficial layers were unaffected in the AD cases. The calbindin-immunoreactive pyramidal neurons of layers III were dramatically affected (up to 60%, Fig. 8) in the disease. Moreover, there was a strong correlation between the extent of the loss of the affected neurons and neurofibrillary tangle counts.

Conclusions

Although regional specialization is a dominant organizational principle for neocortex in all mammalian brains, segregation of functions reaches an extraordinary level of sophistication in primate cortex. Cohesive, integrated processing in a given sensory modality such as vision involves the simultaneous activity of numerous separable visual areas that have extensive, highly ordered interconnections that establish a distributed system subserving vision. Higher intellectual functions, such as cognition and language, that transcend modality-specificity are presumably even more dependent upon the complex communication between cortical regions that is provided by the corticocortical circuits. It is our contention that the long corticocortical projections degenerate in AD, leading to a global neocortical isolation syndrome that is manifested as dementia. Clearly, other degenerative processes occur in AD, and they may also contribute to the behavioral sequelae of AD, but the global loss of long corticocortical projections is likely to be the most devastating component of AD pathology and the most directly related to dementia. Further, the cells that provide these projections appear to be highly specialized neurons that may have identifiable anatomical and biochemical profiles. Combined studies of nonhuman primate and human cortex will be necessary to develop a comprehensive profile of these neurons. We have already initiated such an approach with regard to the morphology, distribution and cytoskeletal profile of these neurons. However, this approach must be extended to include other cytoskeletal elements, growth-associated proteins, growth factor receptors and pre- and postsynaptic markers for specific neurotransmitter systems such as glutamate. If we can pinpoint the elements of the biochemical and anatomical phenotype that are most clearly linked to differential cellular vulnerability in AD, then we will be one step closer to developing means of protecting those neurons that degenerate in AD. The protection of these neurons must be the paramount goal in developing a strategy for the management of AD, since prevention of a neurodegenerative disease is much more likely to be achievable than the development of a cure.

Acknowledgments. We thank T. A. Kimber, R. Guntern, M. Surini, B. Greggio, and S. Hernandez for skillful technical and secretarial assistance. Drs J. Rogers and R. Nakamura provided some of the human postmortem materials used in these studies. Dr. M. R. Celio generously provided the monoclonal antibodies against calcium-binding proteins. This work was supported by grants from the Alzheimer's Disease and Related Disorders Association, the MacArthur Foundation, and NIA (AG06647) to JHM. PRH was the recipient of a fellowship from the Fonds National Suisse de la Recherche Scientifique No. 83.495.0.87.

References

Barbas H (1986) Pattern in the laminar origin of corticocortical connections. J Comp Neurol 252:415–422

Braak H, Braak E (1986) Ratio of pyramidal cells versus non-pyramidal cells in the human frontal isocortex and changes in ratio with ageing and Alzheimer's disease. In: Swaab DF, Fliers E, Mirmiran M, Van Gool WA, Van Haaren F (eds) Progress in Brain Research, vol 70. Elsevier, Amsterdam, pp 185–212

Braak H, Braak E, Kalus P (1989) Alzheimer's disease: areal and laminar pathology in the occipital isocortex. Acta Neuropathol 77:494–506

Campbell MJ, Morrison JH (1989) A monoclonal antibody to neurofilament protein (SMI-32) labels a subpopulation of pyramidal neurons in the human and monkey neocortex. J Comp Neurol 282:191–205

Campbell MJ, Hof PR, Cox K, Timber TA, Young WG, Morrison JH (1989) A subset of primate corticocortical neurons are neurofilament protein (NFP) immunoreactive (ir): a combined retrograde immunohistochemical study. Proc Soc Neurosci 15:72

Celio MR, Schärer L, Morrison JH, Norman AW, Bloom FE (1986) Calbindin immunoreactivity alternates with cytochrome c-oxidase-rich zones in some layers of the primate visual cortex. Nature 323:715–717

Celio MR, Baier W, Schärer L, De Viragh PA, Gerday C (1988) Monoclonal antibodies directed against the calcium binding protein parvalbumin. Cell Calcium 9:81–86

Collerton D (1986) Cholinergic function and intellectual decline in Alzheimer's disease. Neuroscience 19:1–28

Conti F, Fabri M, Manzoni T (1988) Immunocytochemical evidence for glutamatergic corticocortical connections in monkeys. Brain Res 462:148–153

De Lima AD, Voigt T, Morrison JH (1989) Morphology of the cells within the inferior temporal gyrus that project to the prefrontal cortex in the macaque monkey. J Comp Neurol, in press

De Yoe EA, Van Essen DC (1988) Concurrent processing streams in monkey visual cortex. Trends Neurosci 11:219–226

Duyckaerts C, Hauw J-J, Bastenaire F, Piette F, Poulain C, Rainsard V, Javoy-Agid F, Berthaux P (1986) Laminar distribution of neocortical senile plaques in senile dementia of the Alzheimer type. Acta Neuropathol 70:249–256

Greenamyre JT, Penney JB, Young AB, D'Amato CJ, Hicks SP, Shoulson I (1985) Alterations in L-glutamate binding in Alzheimer's and Huntington's diseases. Science 227:1496–1499

Grundke-Iqbal I, Iqbal K, Tung YC, Kinlan M, Wisniewski HM, Binder LI (1986) Abnormal phosphorylation of the microtubule-associated protein (tau) in Alzheimer cytoskeletal pathology. Proc Natl Acad Sci USA 83:4913–4917

Hansen LA, DeTeresa R, Davies P, Terry RD (1988) Neocortical morphometry, lesions counts, and choline acetyltransferase levels in the age spectrum of Alzheimer's disease. Neurology 38:48–54

Hausser CO, Robert F, Giard N (1980) Balint's syndrome. Can J Neurol Sci 7:157–161

Hendry SHC, Jones EG, Emson PC, Lawson DEM, Heizmann CW, Streit P (1989) Two classes of cortical GABA neurons defined by differential calcium binding protein immunoreactivities. Exp Brain Res 767:467–472

Hof PR, Cox K, Morrison JH (1988) Quantitative analysis of non-phosphorylated neurofilament protein (NPNFP)-immunoreactive neurons in normal and Alzheimer's disease brain. Proc Soc Neurosci 14:1086

Hof PR, Bouras C, Constantinidis J, Morrison JH (1989) Balint's syndrome in Alzheimer's disease: specific disruption of the occipito-parietal visual pathway. Brain Res 493:368–375

Hof PR, Bouras C, Constantinidis J, Morrison JH (1989) Selective disconnection of specific visual association pathways in cases of Alzheimer's disease presenting with Balint's syndrome. J Neuropathol Exp Neurol, in press

Hyman BT, Van Hoesen GW, Kromer LJ, Damasio AR (1986) Perforant pathway changes in the memory impairment of Alzheimer's disease. Ann Neurol 20:472–481

Hyman BT, Van Hoesen GW, Damasio AR (1987) Alzheimer's disease: glutamate depletion in the hippocampal perforant pathway zone. Ann Neurol 22:37–40

Iversen LL, Rossor MN, Reynolds GP, Hills R, Roth M, Mountjoy CQ, Foote SL, Morrison JH, Bloom FE (1983) Loss of pigmented dopamine-β-hydroxylase positive cells from locus coeruleus in senile dementia of Alzheimer's type. Neurosci Lett 39:95–100

Joachim CL, Morris JH, Selkoe DJ, Kosik KS (1987) Tau epitopes are incorporated into a range of lesions in Alzheimer's disease. J Neuropathol Exp Neurol 46:611–622

Katz B, Rimmer S (1989) Ophthalmologic manifestations of Alzheimer's disease. Surv Ophthalmol 34:31–43

Kemper TL (1984) Neuroanatomical and neuropathological changes in normal aging and dementia. In: Albert ML (ed) Clinical neurology of aging. Oxford University Press, New York, pp 9–52

Lee VMY, Otvos Jr L, Carden MJ, Hollosi M, Dietzschold B, Lazzarini RA (1988) Identification of the major multiphosphorylation site in mammalian neurofilaments. Proc Natl Acad Sci USA 85:1998–2002

Lewis DA, Campbell MJ, Terry RD, Morrison JH (1987) Laminar and regional distributions of neurofibrillary tangles and neuritic plaques in Alzheimer's disease: a quantitative study of visual and auditory cortices. J Neurosci 7:1799–1808

Mishkin M, Ungerleider LG, Macko KA (1983) Object vision and spatial vision: two cortical pathways. TINS 6:414–417

Morrison JH, Scherr S, Lewis DA, Campbell MJ, Bloom FE, Rogers J, Benoît R (1986) The laminar and regional distribution of neocortical somatostatin and neuritic plaques: implications for Alzheimer's disease as a global neocortical disconnection syndrome. In: Scheibel AB, Wechsler AF (eds) The biological substrates of Alzheimer's disease, UCLA Forum in Medical Sciences, vol 27. Academic, Orlando, pp 115–131

Morrison JH, Lewis DA, Campbell MJ, Huntley GW, Benson DL, Bouras C (1987) A monoclonal antibody to non-phosphorylated neurofilament protein marks the vulnerable cortical neurons in Alzheimer's disease. Brain Res 416:331–336

Morrison JH, Cox K, Hof PR, Celio MR (1988) Neocortical parvalbumin-containing neurons are resistant to degeneration in Alzheimer's disease. Proc Soc Neurosci 14:1085

Mountjoy CQ, Roth M, Evans NJR, Evans HM (1983) Cortical neuronal counts in normal elderly controls and demented patients. Neurobiol Aging 4:1–11

Pearson RCA, Esiri MM, Hiorns RW, Wilcock GK, Powell TPS (1985) Anatomical correlates of the distribution of the pathological changes in the neocortex in Alzheimer disease. Proc Natl Acad Sci USA 82:4531–4534

Perry G, Rizzuto N, Autilio-Gambetti L, Gambetti P (1985) Paired helical filaments from Alzheimer disease patients contain cytoskeletal components. Proc Natl Acad Sci USA 82:3916–3920

Rapoport SI (1987) Alzheimer's disease: phylogenetic vulnerability of associative neocortex and its connections. In: Davies P, Finch CE (eds) Molecular neuropathology of aging, Banbury Report, vol 27. Cold Spring Harbor Laboratory, New York, pp 37–54

Roberts GW, Crow TJ, Polak JM (1985) Location of neuronal tangles in somatostatin neurones in Alzheimer's disease. Nature 314:92–94

Rogers J, Morrison JH (1985) Quantitative morphology and regional and laminar distributions of senile plaques in Alzheimer's disease. J Neurosci 5:2801–2808

Rossor MN (1982) Dementia. Lancet 2:1200–1204

Rossor MN, Iversen LL, Reynolds GP, Mountjoy CQ, Roth M (1984) Neurochemical characteristics of early and late onset types of Alzheimer's disease. Br Med J 288:961–964

Selkoe DJ (1989) Biochemistry of altered brain proteins in Alzheimer's disease. Annu Rev Neurosci 12:463–490

Shipp S, Zeki S (1989a) The organization of connections between areas V5 and V1 in macaque monkey visual cortex. Eur J Neurosci 1:309–332

Shipp S, Zeki S (1989b) The organization of connections between areas V5 and V2 in macaque monkey visual cortex. Eur J Neurosci 1:333–354

Sternberger LA, Sternberger NH (1983) Monoclonal antibodies distinguish phosphorylated and nonphosphorylated forms of neurofilaments in situ. Proc Natl Acad Sci USA 80:6126–6130

Terry RD, Peck A, DeTeresa R, Schechter R, Horoupian DS (1981) Some morphometric aspects of the brain in the senile dementia of the Alzheimer type. Ann Neurol 10:184–192

Van Essen DC (1985) Functional organization of primate visual cortex. In: Peters A, Jones EG (eds) Cerebral cortex, vol 3 (Visual cortex). Plenum Press, New York, pp 259–329

Wilcock GK, Esiri MM (1982) Plaques, tangles and dementia – a quantitative study. J Neurol Sci 56:343–356

Distribution of Neurochemical Deficits in Alzheimer's Disease

*D. M. Bowen, A. J. Cross, P. T. Francis, A. R. Green, S. L. Lowe,
A. W. Procter, J. E. Steele, and G. C. Stratmann*

Summary

Cortical inhibitory neurotransmitters, neuropeptides, dopamine and probably
noradrenaline are probably either not selectively or not critically affected in
Alzheimer's disease. It is, however, highly likely that shrinkage or loss of corticocortical pyramidal neurones is a key change. This change appears to be circumscribed and clinically relevant and to involve neurotransmitter glutamate. The
putative pathogenic role of glutamate is briefly discussed.

Introduction

Alzheimer's disease (AD) has often been approached optimistically as purely a
genetic disorder involving chromosome 21, yet recent research fails to establish
this conclusion for late-onset families (Pericak-Vance et al. 1988). It is generally
accepted that there is a role for genes in the pathogenesis of AD, but a broader
view is necessary because of the strong possibility that the clinical syndrome is a
result of a series of different events over a long period (Bowen et al. 1988). While
AD is a progressive disorder, this fact is rarely acknowledged in the interpretation
of postmortem biochemical studies. Many neurotransmitters have been reported
to be affected, leading some to the pessimistic conclusion that a successful neuro-
transmitter-based therapy will not evolve (Martin et al. 1988). It is argued herein,
however, that dysfunction of a glutamatergic neurotransmitter system is critical.
We seek to link this with perturbations of energy metabolism, a proposed patho-
geneic mechanism, which itself may be "triggered" by an environmental factor,
such as an infectious agent (Pearson and Powell, 1989) or exposure to aluminium
(Candy et al. 1988; but see also Wisniewski et al. 1989). Energy metabolism
cannot be studied with routine postmortem material. The present review, therefore, emphasizes data for transmitters and indices of energy metabolism determined in neurosurgical samples that were obtained soon after the emergence of
symptoms of the disease.

Preserved inhibitory cortical neurotransmitters

Postmortem assessment of these inhibitory cortical neurotransmitters, principally gamma-aminobutyric acid (GABA)-releasing neurones, has been complicated by *artefact and epiphenomena* (as reviewed in Lowe et al. 1988). Thus, no change in glutamate decarboxylase activity was found in a recent study in which AD and control subjects were carefully matched for agonal state (Reinikainen et al. 1988). Tissue atrophy is another factor which may confound interpretation of data. This is because the practice of reporting results relative to unit mass does not make allowance for any reduction in volume of brain structure. Shrinkage or loss of some structures, but not others, may lead to the reporting of an increase in the markers of unaffected structures, such as increased GABA content of frontal cortex from AD biopsy tissue (Lowe et al. 1988). The reductions found in GABA content of most postmortem series are less substantial and widespread than those reported for a group of subjects that included only pathologically severe examples of the disease. Large and widespread reductions in uptake sites of GABAergic neurones have also been reported postmortem. However, since this study was based upon active uptake determinations in tissue that had been frozen, thawed and subfractionated, it is difficult to exclude the possibility that inappropriate preparations were produced in disease-affected tissue. Indeed, others found preservation of this uptake site (assayed using a ligand binding technique) in all regions examined, except the temporal cortex. Moreover, glutamate decarboxylase activity and GABA content of cortical biopsy tissue were not reduced (as reviewed in Lowe et al. 1988, Fig. 1) and an attempt at treating AD with a GABA agonist was unsuccessful (Mohr et al. 1986).

Glycine and taurine are also thought to function as inhibitory neurotransmitters and their content is unchanged in AD, based on both postmortem and biopsy tissue (as reviewed in Lowe et al. 1989). Most enquiries indicate, therefore, that in AD cortical inhibitory neurones are neither selectively nor critically affected.

Preserved Cortical Peptides

Despite relatively high concentrations in cerebral cortex, cholecystokinin, vasoactive intestinal polypeptide and neuropeptide Y are unaffected, as is galanin (Beal et al. 1988). Many studies have demonstrated reduced somatostatin but *not* in biopsy samples (Fig. 1), and there is postmortem evidence of reduced corticotropin-releasing factor (De Souza et al. 1986; but see also Kelley and Kowall 1989). Changes in somatostatin have been found to be greater in studies in which only subjects displaying severe histopathology were examined than in studies in which no such selection criteria were employed (Lowe et al. 1988). A difference in selection criteria may also explain why Beal et al. (1986) found reduced concentrations of neuropeptide Y whereas other groups have reported no change.

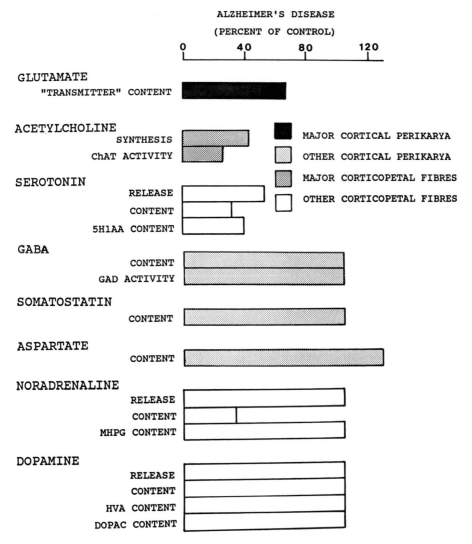

Fig. 1. Selective neurotransmitter changes antemortem: summary of neurotransmitter measures assessed in neocortex of patients with AD. Non-significance is identified by 100% of control (Francis and Bowen 1989; Lowe et al., submitted)

Preservation of Some Corticopetal Neurones

Postmortem Studies

Evidence for presynaptic cholinergic dysfunction in the cerebral cortex in AD has been obtained in all postmortem studies that have measured choline acetyltransferase (ChAT) activity, together with studies of radiolabelled choline uptake and acetylcholine content and release (as reviewed in Francis and Bowen 1989). These data are supported by a myriad of histological studies which have reported loss of cholinergic perikarya from the medial forebrain nucleus basalis of Meynert. Loss of ChAT activity appears to parallel the distribution of neurofibrillary degeneration (tangles) within various cortical areas (Esiri et al. 1989).

With the exception of studies of the serotonin (5-HT) carrier, all estimates of serotonergic neurones in postmortem samples have relied upon determination of the concentrations of 5-HT and its major metabolite, 5-hydroxyindoleacetic acid (5-HIAA). The 5-HT content in the neocortex from AD subjects has, in general, been found to be reduced, whereas 5-HIAA was unaltered except for two reports of a reduced content. There is some evidence from histopathological measurements to indicate that intrinsic cortical change and serotonergic denervation are related, since significant negative correlations were found between neurofibrillary tangle counts and 5-HIAA content in both frontal and temporal cortex of AD subjects. Similarly, the reduction in the concentration of 5-HT is greatest in cortical areas with the most tangles. There is an unexpectedly large reduction in the frontal cortex that appears to be related to aggressive behaviour, suggesting that treatment with serotonomimetic agents could reduce the need for hospitalization (Palmer et al. 1988).

Apart from two studies of dopamine-beta-hydroxylase activity postmortem – one indicating reduced activity and the other finding no change – biochemical studies of catecholaminergic neurones have focussed upon the determination of the concentrations of dopamine and noradrenaline and their principal metabolites, homovanillic acid (HVA) and 3-methoxy-4-hydroxyphenylglycol (MHPG), respectively. The concentration of dopamine has consistently been found not to be reduced. HVA concentrations are reported to be reduced in some regions but elevated in others. Reduced concentrations of noradrenaline have generally been reported, whereas concentrations of MHPG have been reported as reduced, unaltered or even elevated.

Antemortem Studies

Small amounts of AD brain tissue, removed for diagnostic purposes, have also been used for biochemical analyses, an approach pioneered by Korey et al. (1961). Only a few samples have been offered to our laboratory (39 from seven centres, between 1976 and 1987), yet these have been extremely useful. We have shown that severe cholinergic and serotonergic deficiencies occur within 2–3 years of onset of symptoms (Fig. 1). The sparing of catecholamines and the association between 5-HIAA content and tangle count have been confirmed. Detailed clinico-pathological assessments have been made, including a rating of the magnitude of dementia on the basis of the performance of patients on a number of tests that assessed the extent of the following clinical domains: memory, perceptuo-spatial abilities and language. The rating correlated with acetylcholine synthesis (Francis et al. 1985) but not with other corticopetal transmitters (Palmer et al. 1987).

Degeneration of Corticocortical Association Fibers

From results of a number of histological and positron emission tomographic (PET) enquiries, degeneration of corticocortical association fibres appears to be a feature of AD. Firstly, degeneration of these fibres in AD is indicated by loss of columns of pyramidal neurones, based on a shorter cortical ribbon and the distribution of tangles and senile plaques (as reviewed in Procter et al. 1988, 1989a). Secondly, loss of neurones giving rise to association fibres appears to occur relatively early in the disease, as pyramidal cell counts (corrected for any cortical thinning) are reduced in cortical layer III of biopsy tissue from the temporal lobe (Neary et al. 1986). Thirdly, shrinkage and loss of pyramidal neurones from the temporal and parietal lobes may be the major cause of cerebral atrophy in AD. When studied by PET these regions show apparent glucose hypometabolism; measurements by this technique are sensitive to atrophy, and hypometabolism is not seen in vitro (Table 1). Thus, scanning results may actually index, in part, the early shrinkage or loss of pyramidal cells giving rise to corticocortical association fibres. Neuropsychological test scores significantly correlate with both scanning data (as reviewed in Procter et al. 1989a) and pyramidal cell counts in layer III (Neary et al. 1986). In summary, it is highly probable that shrinkage or loss of association fibres occurs from circumscribed areas, mainly the temporal and parietal lobes. Moreover, this change appears to be clinically relevant.

Table 1. No evidence for hypometabolism in antemortem samples from patients with AD[a]

Tissue preparation	Marker	Marker in samples from AD patients (% of control)
Cerebral cortex, homogenates	Oxygen uptake	
	+ADP $(n=5, 7)$[b]	120
	−ADP $(n=5, 7)$	181 *
	+CCC[c] $(n=5, 7)$	102
Cerebral cortex, tissue prisms	[U-^{14}C]glucose → $^{14}CO_2$	
	5 mMK$^+$ $(n= 9, 17)$[b]	142 **
	31 MMK$^+$ $(n=22, 27)$	128 **
Skin fibroblasts, confluent monolayers	[U-^{14}C]glucose → $^{14}CO_2$ $(n=6, 7)$	128 **
	Lactate release $(n=6, 7)$	118 *

[a] Data from Sims et al. (1981, 1983, 1985, 1987a,b)
[b] Values in parentheses are the number of independent samples studied for AD patients and controls, respectively
[c] CCCP, carbonyl cyanide *m*-chlorophenylhydrazone, an uncoupling agent. * $p<0.05$; ** $p<0.001$ significantly different from control

Excitatory Dicarboxylic Amino Acids (EDAAs) Are Probably Transmitters of Pyramidal Neurones Forming Corticocortical Association Fibres

Although quantitative electron microscopic data indicate that pyramidal cells constitute the most abundant neuronal type in the mammalian neocortex, the transmitter(s) associated with this cell type has not been established unequivocally. Major candidates are EDAAs, principally L-aspartate and L-glutamate. There is a variety of evidence for this, largely from studies of the corticostriatal pathway. The possibility of corticocortical glutamatergic pathways is particularly difficult to establish, in part because a technique has not been developed for destroying pyramidal neurones selectively in the cerebral cortex of experimental animals. Human as well as rat cerebral cortex has a high-affinity uptake system for the false EDAA transmitter, D-aspartate, and shows Ca^{2+}-dependent K^+-stimulated release of aspartate and glutamate (see Peinado and Mora 1986; Procter et al. 1988). These glutamatergic terminals could be thalamocortical projections, the other major source of excitatory cortical fibres. However, thalamic pathology in AD is less prominent than cortical changes. D-[^{3}h] Aspartate uptake is reduced by 50% in temporal cortex from promptly performed autopsies of AD patients, using a technique designed to minimize influences of artefacts and epiphenomena (Procter et al. 1988). This provides evidence that a large proportion of the glutamatergic terminals in the cerebral cortex are in fact synapses of corticocortical fibres. Glutamate content of the grey matter from biopsy samples of AD patients is also reduced (Procter et al. 1988) and the value for individual subjects correlates with pyramidal neurone density in layer III (Lowe et al., submitted). The most straightforward explanation is that loss of corticocortical association fibres has had a major influence on the glutamate content of these samples. In summary, these results provide new evidence that an EDAA, probably L-glutamate, is the principal transmitter of corticocortical association fibres.

Excitatory Dicarboxylic Amino Acid Neurotransmission and Magnitude of Dementia

No study has so far been reported that seeks to directly relate an index of glutamatergic neurotransmission of the magnitude of dementia. There is, however, evidence that EDAA neurotransmitter dysfunction relates to memory and behavioural disturbance. Firstly, such dysfunction may be prominent in critical structures, the hippocampus (Hyman et al. 1987) and amygdala (Francis et al. 1987). Secondly, histological and PET enquiries, loss of tissue glutamate and reduced D-aspartate uptake suggest that, in AD, degeneration occurs in a proportion of glutamatergic corticocortical neurones and, as has already been argued, is clinically relevant. Thirdly, the presence in the cortex of pyramidal cells with synaptic targets of other pyramidal neurones, and the abundance therein of both L-glutamate binding sites and pyramidal cells, suggests that EDAA neurotransmission is normally the major factor that sustains the activity of corticocortical neurones (Peinado and Mora 1986; Procter et al. 1989a). Finally, the primary agonist site of the N-methyl-D-aspartate (NMDA) receptor complex is the best characterized binding site for L-glutamate, and animal studies implicate the complex in memory and behaviour (i.e., experience-dependent changes in kitten visual cortex, initiation of long-term potentiation, acquisition of place learning in rodents and storage of information during learning in chicks; as reviewed in McCabe and Horn 1988).

Although altered populations of recognition sites for EDAAs have been reported for AD in the neostriatum and the hippocampus, the neocortex has shown few alterations. Lower glutamate binding in cortical layers 1 and 2 (with an autoradiographic technique) and reduced glycine modulation of the NMDA receptor complex have been described (as reviewed in Procter et al. 1989b). However, a number of properties of the complex remain unchanged, including the primary agonist (i.e., glutamate) recognition site (with a technique using well-washed membranes), suggesting that pharmacological manipulation of the glycine modulatory domain (Procter et al. 1989a; Steele et al. 1989a) may provide an approach for restoring the activity of the remaining pyramidal neurones.

Neurotransmitter-Based Treatment Strategy

Alzheimer's disease is a fatal disorder with widespread social and economic implications, so a therapy is urgently required. In addition to the cholinergic deficit, a proportion of the glutamatergic corticocortical neurones in the temporal and parietal lobes that probably receive an extensive EDAA input seem to degenerate in AD. Various pharmacological paradigms related to EDAA neurotransmission have been shown, in rodents, to be modified both in vivo and in vitro by tetrahydro-9-aminoacridine. These effects are only observed with high concentrations. Therefore, if tacrine is efficacious in AD patients, it is likely to be through brain cholinergic systems rather than via EDAA systems (Steele et al. 1989b).

Does glutamatergic dysfunction cause changes in memory and behaviour? Can the activity of the remaining neurones be safely restored with a drug active towards the NMDA-receptor complex? Will this provide clinical benefit? These questions cannot be answered without further research, but a glycine modulatory domain of the NMDA receptor complex has already been described at which potential therapeutic agents might be directed. Safety, the extent of occupancy of the modulatory domain by glycine and any other endogenous compounds, influence of other classes of EDAA receptors, as well as the magnitude of neuronal loss are important factors that will determine whether this therapeutic approach will be successful.

Metabolism and EDAAs

A widely documented change in the brains of patients with AD is an apparent reduction in cerebral metabolism, based on blood flow and the metabolic rate for oxygen (as reviewed in Gustafson et al. 1987; Najlerahim and Bowen 1988) as well as for glucose, as described above. Studies of postmortem AD brains also indicate reduced activities of enzymes of carbohydrate metabolism including aldolase, phosphohexoseisomerase and phosphoglycerate mutase (as reviewed in Bowen and Davison 1986). However, these data need to be interpreted with caution as measurements by in vivo imaging techniques may reflect a combination of cortical atrophy, loss of "activating reticular" (corticopetal) innervation and disproportionately more inhibitory neurones, in addition to an intrinsic metabolic dysfunction of cortical neurones (as reviewed in Chawluk et al. 1987; Najlerahim and Bowen 1988). Moreover, it is difficult to completely rule out complicating effects of perimortem hypoxic changes on the enzymes in postmortem brain (Sims et al. 1987a). Indeed, studies of biopsy tissue (Table 1) have shown that the oxidative capacity of brain tissue from AD patients may actually be increased. This has been interpreted as reflecting a partial uncoupling of mitochondria or an increased basal metabolic activity as a consequence of neuronal degeneration and reactive gliosis (Sims et al. 1987a). Electron microscopic studies of cortical biopsies of AD patients have revealed structural abnormalities in mitochondria of otherwise normal dendrites (Savaura et al. 1985) and a reduced volume of tangle-bearing perikaryal cytoplasm per mitochondrion (Sumpter et al. 1986). There is also evidence of altered glucose metabolism in some non-neuronal tissues from AD patients, including fibroblasts (Table 1). It is becoming increasingly apparent that skin and nasal epithelium demonstrate other pathological features of AD brains and could provide not only a non-invasive diagnostic tool but prove pivotal for the investigation of pathogenic mechanisms (Joachim et al. 1989; Talamo et al. 1989). For example, a study of fibroblasts suggests that AD is a disorder in which a pathologically low intracellular calcium content occurs (Peterson et al. 1986) and "down-regulation" (Procter et al. 1989a, b) of the NMDA receptor complex-operated calcium channel (Siesjo and Bengtsson 1989) may reduce this further within vulnerable pyramidal cells. Calcium activates pyruvate dehydrogenase (Hansford and Castro 1985; Moreno-Sanchez and Hansford 1988) and in AD the enzyme has been reported to be reduced (as reviewed in Sorbi et al. 1983). This scheme provides a further mechanism which may lead to perturbations of neuronal energy metabolism. A consequence of the latter might be the transition of endogenous NMDA agonists (e.g., glutamate) from transmitters to neurotoxins (as reviewed in Henneberry 1989). Mechanisms involving the NMDA receptor complex that may render subpopulations of neurones particularly vulnerable to these neurotoxins have been proposed (Greenamyre and Young 1989; Siesjo and Bengtsson 1989). Further research is required to advance these proposals beyond speculation. The evidence herein indicates that a proportion of cortical EDAA-releasing pyramidal neurones degenerate. Is this due to excitotoxicity and will NMDA agonists act as "cognitive enhancers?"

Acknowledgements. Supported in part by the Brain Research Trust ("Miriam Marks Department").

References

Beal MF, Clevens RA, Chattha GK, MacGarvey MU, Mazurek MF, Gabriel SM (1986) Neuropeptide Y immunoreactivity is reduced in cerebral cortex in Alzheimer's disease. Ann Neurol 20:282–288

Beal MF, Clevens RA, Chattha GK, MacGarvey MU, Mazurek MF, Gabriel SM (1988) Galanin-like immunoreactivity is unchanged in Alzheimer's disease and Parkinson's disease. J Neurochem 51:1935–1941

Bowen DM, Davison AN (1986) Biochemical studies of nerve cells and energy metabolism in Alzheimer's disease. Br Med Bull 42:75–80

Bowen DM, Beyreuther K, Cross AJ, Davies P, Diringer H, Goldgaber D, Hock FJ, Khachaturian ZS, Kurz AF, Masters CL, Multhaup G, Price DL, Saper CB (1988) Group report. Cell injury: molecular biology and genetic basis. In: Henderson AS, Henderson JH (eds) Etiology of dementia of Alzheimer's type. Wiley, Chichester, pp 165–176

Candy J, Oakley A, Gauvreau D, Chalker P, Bishop H, Moon D, Staines G, Edwardson J (1988) Association of aluminium and silicon with neuropathological changes in the ageing brain. In: Von Hahn HP (ed) Interdiscipl Topics Geront Vol 25. Karger, Basel, pp 140–155

Chawluk JB, Alavi A, Dann R, Hurlig HI, Bais S, Kushner M, Zimmerman RA, Reivich MJ (1987) Positron emission tomography in aging and dementia: effect of cerebral atrophy. J Nucl Med 28:431–437

De Souza EB, Whitehouse PJ, Kuhor MJ, Price DC, Vale WW (1986) Reciprocal changes in corticotropin releasing factor (CRF)-like immunoreactivity and CRF receptors in cerebral cortex of Alzheimer's disease. Nature 319:539–545

Esiri MM, Pearson RCA, Steele JE, Bowen DM, Powell TPS (1989) A quantitative study of the neurofibrillary tangles and the choline acetyltransferase activity in the cerebral cortex and the amygdala in Alzheimer's disease. J Neurol Neurosurg Psychiat in press

Francis PT, Bowen DM (1989) Tacrine, a drug with therapeutic potential for dementia: postmortem biochemical evidence. Can J Neurol Sci, 16:504–510

Francis PT, Palmer AM, Sims NR, Bowen DM, Davison AN, Esiri MM, Neary D, Snowden JS, Wilcock GK (1985) Neurochemical studies of early-onset Alzheimer's disease: possible influence on treatment. N Engl J Med 313:7–11

Francis PT, Pearson RCA, Lowe SL, Neal JN, Stephens PH, Powell TPS, Bowen DM (1987) The dementia of Alzheimer's disease: an update. J Neurol Neurosurg Psychiat 50:242–243

Greenamyre JT, Young AB (1989) Author's response to commentaries. Neurobiol Aging 10:618–620

Gustafson L, Edvinson L, Dahlgren N, Hagberg B, Risberg J, Rosen I, Ferno H (1987) Intravenous physostigmine treatment of Alzheimer's disease evaluated by psychometric testing, regional cerebral blood flow (rCBF) measurement, and EEG. Psychopharmacology 93:31–35

Hansford RG, Castro F (1985) Role of Ca^{2+} in pyruvate dehydrogenase interconversion in brain mitochondria and synaptosomes. Biochem J 227:129–136

Henneberry RG (1989) The role of neuronal energy in the neurotoxicity of excitatory amino acids. Neurobiol Aging 10:611–613

Hyman BT, Van Hoesen GW, Damansio AR (1987) Alzheimer's disease: glutamate depletion in hippocampal perforant pathway zone. Ann Neurol 22:37–40

Joachim CL, Mori H, Selkoe DJ (1989) Amyloid β-protein deposition in tissue other than brain in Alzheimer's disease. Nature 341:226–230

Kelley M, Kowall N (1989) Corticotropin-releasing factor immunoreactive neurons persist throughout the brain in Alzheimer's disease. Brain Res 501:392–396

Korey SR, Scheinberg L, Terry R, Stein A (1961) Studies in presenile dementon. Trans Am Neurol Assoc 86:99–102

Lowe SL, Francis PT, Procter AW, Palmer AM, Davison AN, Bowen DM (1988) Gamma-aminobutyric acid concentration in brain tissue at two stages of Alzheimer's disease. Brain 111:785–799

Martin JB, Beal MF, Mazurek M, Kowall NW, Growdon JH (1988) Some observations on the significance of neurotransmitter changes in Alzheimer's disease. In: Terry RD (ed) Aging and the brain. Aging Vol 32. Raven, New York, pp 129–148

McCabe BJ, Horn G (1988) Learning and memory; regional changes in N-methyl-D-aspartate receptors in the chick brain. Proc Natl Acad Sci USA 85:2849–2855

Mohr E, Bruno G, Foster N, Gillespie M, Cox C, Hare TA, Tamminga C, Fedio P, Chase TN (1986) GABA-agonist therapy for Alzheimer's disease. Clin Neuropharmacol 9:257–263

Moreno-Sanchez R, Hansford RC (1988) Dependence of cardiac mitochondrial pyruvate dehydrogenase activity on intramitochondrial free Ca^{2+} concentration. Biochem J 256:403–412

Najlerahim A, Bowen DM (1988) Biochemical measurements in Alzheimer's disease reveal a necessity for improved neuroimaging techniques to study metabolism. Biochem J 251:305–308

Neary D, Snowden JS, Mann DMA, Northern B, Bowen DM, Sims NR, Yates PO, Davison AN (1986) Alzheimer's disease: a correlative study. J Neurol Neurosurg Psychiat 49:229–237

Palmer AM, Francis PT, Bowen DM, Benton JS, Neary D, Mann DMA, Snowden JS (1987) Catecholaminergic neurones assessed antimortem in Alzheimer's disease. Brain Res 414:365–370

Palmer AM, Stratmann GC, Procter AW, Bowen DM (1988) Possible neurotransmitter basis of behavioural changes in Alzheimer's disease. Ann Neurol 23:616–620

Pearson RCA, Powell TPS (1989) The neuroanatomy of Alzheimer's disease. Rev Neurosci, in press

Peinado JM, Mora F (1986) Glutamic acid as putative transmitter of the interhemispheric corticocortical connections in the rat. J Neurochem 47:1598–1603

Pericak-Vance MA, Yamaoka LH, Haynes CS, Speer MC, Haines JL, Gaskell PC, Hung W-Y, Clark CM, Heyman AL, Trofatter JA, Eisenmenger JP, Gilbert JR, Lee JE, Alberts MJ, Dawson DV, Bartlett RJ, Earl NL, Siddique T, Vance JM, Conneally PM, Roses AD (1988) Genetic linkage studies in Alzheimer's disease families. Exp Neurol 102:271–279

Peterson C, Ratan RR, Shelanski ML, Goldman JE (1986) Cytosolic free calcium and cell spreading decrease in fibroblasts from aged and Alzheimer donors. Proc Natl Acad Sci USA 83:7999–8001

Procter AW, Palmer AM, Francis PT, Lowe SL, Neary D, Murphy E, Doshi R, Bowen DM (1988) Evidence of glutamatergic denervation and possible abnormal metabolism in Alzheimer's disease. J Neurochem 50:790–802

Procter AW, Wong EHF, Stratmann GC, Lowe SL, Bowen DM (1989a) Reduced glycine stimulation of [^{3}H] MK801 binding in Alzheimer's disease. J Neurochem 53:698–704

Procter AW, Stirling JM, Stratmann GC, Cross AJ, Bowen DM (1989b) Loss of glycine-dependent radioligand binding to the N-methyl-D-aspartate-phencyclidine receptor complex in patients with Alzheimer's disease. Iveroscie Lett 101:62–66

Reinikainen KJ, Paljarvi L, Huuskonen M, Soininen H, Laakso M, Riekkinen PJ (1988) A postmortem study of noradrenergic serotonergic and GABAergic neurones in Alzheimer's disease. J Neurol Sci 84:101–116

Savaura AA, Borges MM, Madeira MD, Tavares MA, Paula-Barbosa MM (1985) Mitochondrial abnormalities in cortical dendrites from patients with Alzheimer's disease. J Submicroscop Cytol 17:459–464

Siesjo BK, Bengtsson F (1989) Calcium fluxes, calcium antagonists and calcium-related pathology in brain ischemia, hypoglycemia and spreading depression, a unifying hypothesis. J Cereb Blood Flow Metab 9:127–140

Sims NR, Bowen DM, Davison AN (1981) [^{14}C]Acetylcholine synthesis and [^{14}C]carbon dioxide production from [U^{14}C]glucose by tissue prisms from human neocortex. Biochem J 196:867–876

Sims NR, Bowen DM, Neary D, Davison AN (1983) Metabolic processes in Alzheimer's disease: adenine nucleotide content and production of $^{14}CO_2$ from [U-^{14}C]glucose in vitro in human neocortex. J Neurochem 41:1329–1334

Sims NR, Finegan JM, Blass JP (1985) Altered glucose metabolism in fibroblasts from patients with Alzheimer's disease. N Engl J Med 313:638–639

Sims NR, Finegan JM, Blass JP, Bowen DM, Neary D (1987a) Mitochondrial function in brain tissue in primary degenerative dementia. Brain Res 436:30–38

Sims NR, Finegan JM, Blass JP (1987b) Altered metabolic properties of cultured skin fibroblasts in Alzheimer's disease. Ann Neurol 21:451–457

Sorbi S, Bird ED, Blass JP (1983) Decreased pyruvate dehydrogenase complex activity in Huntington and Alzheimer brain. Ann Neurol 13:72–78

Sumpter PQ, Mann DMA, Davies CA, Yates PO, Snowden JS, Neary D (1986) An ultrastructural analysis of the effects of accumulation of neurofibrillary tangle in pyramidal neurones of the cerebral cortex in Alzheimer's disease. Neuropath Appl Neurobiol 12:305–319

Steele JE, Palmer HM, Stratmann GC, Bowen DM (1989a) The N-methyl-D-aspartate receptor complex in Alzheimer's disease: reduced regulation by glycine but not zinc. Brain Res, in press

Steele JE, Palmer AM, Lowe SI, Bowen DM (1989b) The influence of tetrahydro-9-amino-acridine on excitatory amino acid neurotransmission in vivo and in vitro. Br J Pharmacol 96:353P

Talamo BR, Rudel R, Kosik KS, Lee VMY, Neff S, Adelman L, Kanver JS (1989) Pathological changes in olfactory neurones in patients with Alzheimer's disease. Nature 337:786–793

Wisniewski HM, Moretz RC, Iqbal K (1989) No evidence for aluminium in etiology and pathogenesis of Alzheimer's disease. Neurobiol Aging 532–535

Topography of Lesions in Alzheimer's Disease: A Challenge to Morphologists

J.-J. Hauw, C. Duyckaerts, P. Delaère, and F. Piette

Summary

The distribution of lesions in Alzheimer's disease (AD) is a much more widely debated topic today than it was a few years ago for the following reasons: (1) many epidemiological biases (lack of recognized criteria for normality in aging, frequency of associated pathologies, cohort effects) have been ignored by morphologists using retrospective data; (2) cerebral atrophy could be due mainly to loss of corticosubcortical radial columns of interconnected neurons and associated glial cells and myelin sheaths; (3) as a consequence, the measurement of neurons on histological samples deals mainly with their density and not with their actual number; (4) the density of the various types of lesions of gray matter seen in AD is different from one area to another, and global indexes could be misleading; (4) histochemistry with antibodies to proteins tau, Alz 50, and overall A4 has provided a broader range and a larger distribution of changes; and (5) the evidence concerning the extent and mechanism of white matter lesions is conflicting. The main pertinent data from the literature are critically assessed below.

Introduction

The distribution of lesions in Alzheimer's disease (AD) is more under debate now than it was a few years ago. This is due to the recent burst of research work in morphology of aging and dementias and to the recognition of the numerous pitfalls of early studies.

Biases in the Study of the Neuropathology of AD

A few simple and obvious biases have often been ignored and have introduced a lot of confusion into the data (Hauw et al. 1988, 1989). One of the main difficulties comes from the early recognition that pathological changes observed in AD are qualitatively similar to some of those seen with increasing prevalence and density in so-called normal aging. Thus, the distinction between AD and normal aging of the brain can be difficult, especially in very old patients, with some cases being classified as mild AD or as normal brain as a function of arbitrary criteria. As a matter of fact, normality of an aged brain is difficult to define.

Criteria for Normality

Criteria for normality have not been established or even discussed by most morphologists: which meaning of the word "normal" should be used? Among the seven meanings proposed by Dr. Murphy, four are widely used in medicine and biology: *clinical* (innocuous: for example, corpora amylacea are normal) or *descriptive* (habitual; for example, a few senile plaques in the temporal cortex are normal in the elderly). These meanings are currently used in the diagnosis of individual cases. By contrast, we could use more probabilistic meanings for normality such as the *genetic* sense (i.e., the fittest; for example less than five senile plaques/mm^2 are normal in a 75-year-old woman; more would mean a deviation less suitable for survival, i.e., a disease, namely AD) or the *statistical* meaning (better to say *gaussian,* i.e., to find ten plaques/mm^2 in the same woman is normal, since this plaque density is included in a 95 confidence interval of the whole group of women of this age, whatever their clinical status). Medicine and biology today tend to use the latter meanings for normality, which better fit population and research studies. The use of a gaussian meaning for normality in medicine is open to criticism, since this implies a normal distribution and dismisses the presence of two or more populations, such as normal subjects and patients (Galen and Gambino 1975). The choice between criteria favoring discontinuity or continuity in the concepts of aging and disease is not only a question of philosophy.

Pitfalls for the Study of Normal Aging and AD

Some morphological studies do not fulfill the conditions for exclusion of associated disorders, which are very numerous in the elderly. In addition, other pitfalls such as cohort effects have been ignored for a long time and are, surprisingly, still ignored in some recent studies. It may be recalled, for example, that the comparison of the brain weight of individuals born at a 80-year interval led to overestimation of the brain atrophy of aging. The mean brain weight of people from industrialized countries increased by nearly 100 g over a century, as did body weight and height (Dekaban and Sadowsky 1978; Miller et al. 1980). Prospective studies are the most suitable for avoiding these pitfalls.

Clinical Data, Pathological Data or Both?

Lastly, the diagnosis depends upon the data at hand: when these data are only clinical, the increasing quality of diagnostic criteria is mainly concerned with their specificity. On the contrary, their sensitivity is still poor (Katzman et al. 1988). This leads to the selection of well-contrasted groups of severely affected patients. Cases which are excluded from these studies can be normal or affected by mild

AD (or by other diseases). It is important to stress that the use of normative criteria as specific as those used for AD is mandatory. The level of difficulty is different when dealing only with neuropathological data or with clinical and neuropathological data. A strict clinicopathological point of view is useful since "dementia" is a clinical term (and cannot be diagnosed with certainty by the pathologist) and "AD" is a pathological one (conversely, it cannot be diagnosed with certainty by the clinician). However, in AD clinical abnormalities are linked to the distribution and to the density of morphological changes. The linkage is complex, with threshold effects that may be due in part to our measuring instruments (psychometry as well as morphometrical techniques). As a consequence, the diagnosis of dementia of the Alzheimer type is probabilistic when using only clinical or histological means. The highest degree of probability, i.e., definite AD, is obtained when using both. As another consequence, with some methodological precautions, it should be possible to evaluate the role of individual lesions such as tangles or plaques in causing dementia in AD. The more they are statistically linked to the mental deterioration, the more these lesions are likely to be relevant to this deterioration.

Longitudinal Studies

Since the pioneering work of Blessed et al. (1968), new findings have been obtained from longitudinal studies (Mountjoy et al. 1983; Sulkava et al. 1983; Berg et al. 1984; Terry et al. 1981, 1987; Tierney et al. 1988; Moosy et al. 1989). Eight years ago, we undertook a prospective study (Charles Foix longitudinal study) with the specific aim of searching for links between the mental decline and the main lesions of late-onset AD (senile dementia of the Alzheimer type (SDAT). We studied the pathology of 28 cases from a group of women over 75 living in the same institution. Their mental level had been assessed by the same team, using the test score of Blessed et al. (1968), which was the only neuropathologically validated test at the time this study began. Individuals were either normal or affected by SDAT with varying degrees of severity. This was ascertained by clinical and neuropathological exclusion of every other cause of dementia. Blindness or deafness were additional causes for exclusion since they could disturb the mental evaluation. This choice of noncontrasted groups enabled us to include a whole set of degrees of mental impairment, including mild or moderate – possibly early – cases of AD. This led to a gaussian distribution of mental scores and, in most cases, of lesions.

Cerebral Atrophy

Loss of Brain Weight and Volume

Once the secular increase in brain weight (Miller and Corsellis, 1977) is taken into account, all neuropathological studies, whatever the technique used, indicate a steady and slow decrease in brain weight (2%/decade on average) occurring from 50 years onwards in normal aging, even in carefully selected cases (Davis and Wright 1977; Dekaban and Sadowsky 1978; Miller et al. 1980; Terry et al. 1987).

Grey and White Matter

In normal aging, the ratio of grey to white matter increases from 1.13 in individuals born 50 years ago to 1.55 in centenarians. In SDAT, no change in this ratio has been found (Miller et al. 1980; De la Monte 1989). However, reduction in the volume of white matter during AD has been recently reported by De la Monte (1989) in four preclinical cases, i.e., apparently normal but not prospectively studied persons with numerous senile changes at neuropathology. The description of incomplete white matter infarctions in large proportions of cases of AD by Brun and Englund (1986) has raised some controversies concerning this topic. The pathogenesis (relationship to amyloid angiopathy) and the relevance to pure AD or to mixed dementia (AD plus vascular dementia) of the changes described by these authors remain controversial. As a matter of fact, in mixed dementias, white matter rarefaction, as seen in Binswanger's disease or in amyloid angiopathy, is common. By contrast, it is less conspicuous in pure AD without vascular risk factors. Quantitative studies on the density of myelinated fibers in AD are lacking. Most authors think that the cerebral cortex and some deep nuclei bear the brunt of the lesions and that the white matter changes are secondary.

Cortical Atrophy

In elderly normal individuals, Tomlinson et al. (1968) found no case with marked or generalized gyral atrophy on neuropathological examination. By contrast, it is a frequent feature in AD, being more severe in the early-onset forms than in SDAT. The neocortical surface area of all the cerebral lobes was significantly decreased in early-onset forms of AD, whereas only the temporal lobe was atrophic in cases of SDAT over 80 years' of age (Hubbard and Anderson 1981). It must be emphasized that gyral atrophy is an inconstant feature, even in early-onset AD. It may be asymmetric and predominates in some areas (emphasis has been repeatedly placed on the association areas).

The thickness of the neocortex is only slightly affected by normal aging (Kemper 1984; Hansen et al. 1988). Terry et al. (1987) showed a moderate but significant decrease with age in the midfrontal and superior temporal areas but not in inferior parietal areas. Surprisingly, the decrease in thickness of the neocortex is also moderate in AD and especially in SDAT (for review see Kemper 1984; Hansen et al. 1988). We have proposed that the decrease of the cortical area measured on sections of the brain (i.e., neocortical atrophy) could be mainly due to a decrease in the length of the cortical ribbon when measured on coronal sections, whereas its thickness did not vary significantly at least in the early stages of the disease. A correlation was indeed found between the length – and not the thickness – of the cortical ribbon and mental decline in the Charles Foix longitu-

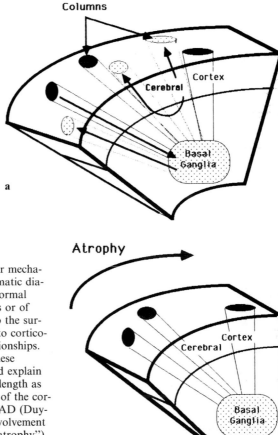

Fig. 1a,b. Mechanism of columnar mechanism for cerebral atrophy. **a** Schematic diagram of the cerebral cortex of a normal brain showing columns of neurons or of fibers, arranged perpendicularly to the surface of the cortex, corresponding to corticocortical or corticosubcortical relationships. **b** Atrophy after loss of some of these columns. Such a mechanism would explain the predominant reduction in the length as compared to that in the thickness of the cortical ribbon in the early stages of AD (Duyckaerts et al. 1985). A selective involvement of some cortical layers ("laminar atrophy") would induce by contrast the predominant reduction in the thickness of the cortex

dinal study (Duyckaerts et al. 1985; Hauw et al. 1987). These data suggest that cortical atrophy is mainly due, at least at the beginning of the disease, to a loss of columns of neurons or of fibers, arranged perpendicularly to the surface of the cortex (Fig. 1). These columns could correspond to the developmental columns studied by Rakic (1988). The loss of selective layers of the neocortex (laminar loss) would instead alter the thickness of the cortical ribbon. The latter is detectable only in the most affected cases, especially in early-onset AD, where it can be seen upon gross examination, especially in the temporal cortex.

Neuronal Loss

Some neuronal loss is easy to measure in small, limited structures such as deep nuclei where it is well established in aging and in AD (Table 1). However, neu-

Table 1. Reported data on neuronal loss in aging and AD

Neuronal loss	Normal aging	SDAT
Neocortex Maximum in temporal and frontal lobes	± (severity and cell type debated) Atrophy of some classes (middle-sized pyramidal neurons)	+ (severity debated) + + Middle-sized pyra- midal neurons
Hippocampus	+ Pyramidal neurons CA 1, etc.	+ + Pyramidal neurons
Amygdala	+ Phylogenetically older areas	+ +
Cingulum	±	+
Basal ganglia	*Variable*	*Variable*
Basal magnocellular complex	+	+ +
Median mammillary nucleus	±	+
Paraventricular and supra- chiasmatic nuclei	(debated; may depend on patient age)	
Brainstem	*Variable*	*Variable*
Locus ceruleus	+	+ +
Substantia nigra	+	+
Cerebellum (Purkinje cells)	+ +	−
Retina (ganglion cells)	?	+ +

Data from: Ball and Lo (1977), Blanks and Blanks (1988), Dam AM (1979), Doebler et al. (1987), Hansen et al. (1988), Herzog and Kemper (1980), Kemper (1984), Mann (1988), Mann et al. (1985), Mountjoy et al. (1983), Swaab et al. (1985), Terry et al. (1981, 1987)

ronal loss has often been overestimated on account of associated atrophy of neuronal cell bodies, which makes them less likely to be cut on histological sections (Duyckaerts et al. 1989 b). In the cerebral cortex, we do not know the precise location and magnitude of neuronal loss.

In the hippocampus, a neuronal loss of around 25% has been recorded by Ball and Lo (1977) and Dam (1979) in normal aging. In AD, the reduction of cell number in the pyramidal layer of the hippocampus reaches 40% – 60% (Ball and Lo 1977; Mann et al. 1985). It predominates in CA1 and in the subiculum, but cytochemical techniques showed that pyramidal neuronal RNA was diffusely reduced in all areas of the hippocampus examined (Doebler et al. 1987). This loss has been found to be highly correlated with the number of tangle-bearing cells (Ball and Lo 1977; Doebler et al. 1987). A marked cell loss is also seen in the entorhinal cortex (Hyman et al. 1988) and in the amygdala (Herzog and Kemper 1980; Mann 1988).

Data concerning the neocortex are very controversial. In normal aging, quantitative data are confusing, but well-controlled recent studies indicate that there is some neuronal atrophy (decrease of the volume of neuronal cell body) and little, if any, neuronal loss (Haug et al. 1984; Meyer-Ruge et al. 1984; Terry et al. 1987). In AD, recent studies have shown a slight reduction in the number of neuronal cell bodies, which is lacking in some areas (Table 2). Only results concerning the temporal cortex can be compared. The morphometric techniques and, overall, the definition of the measured area on the samples examined at the microscopic level were different. Terry et al. (1981) and Hansen et al. (1988) measured the number

Table 2. Reported data on neocortical cell loss in AD[a]

	Frontal (middle)	Temporal (superior)	Parietal (inferior)	Occipital (Brodman 17)	Cingular (Brodman 24)
Terry et al. (1981)[b]	26 (46)*	22 (40)*			
Hansen et al. (1988)					
Young AD (50–65 years)	23 (50)*	26 (44)*	36 (58)*		
Old AD (70–100 years)	18 (27)*	15 (29)*	6 (27)*		
Mountjoy et al. (1983)	12	18	1***	9	11
Mann et al. (1985)**		40 (60)****			

[a] Percentage reduction of neuronal number measured on samples processed for microscopic examination, as compared with age-matched controls: ( ), pyramidal neurons; *, large pyramidal cells ($>90 \mu m^2$); **, data corrected for cortical thickness; ***, superior medial parietal region; ****, middle temporal gyrus.
[b] Terry et al. (1981) and Hansen et al. (1988) used automatic analysis with editing to measure a given length of the cortical ribbon; Mountjoy et al. (1983) used automatic analysis without editing to measure columns perpendicular to the surface of the cortex; Mann et al. (1985) used manual counting with the same procedure and made a correction to take into account the reduction in the thickness of the cortex

of neurons in a given length of the cortical ribbon. Mountjoy et al. (1983) measured the density of neurons in columns perpendicular to the surface of the cortex. Mann et al. (1985) used the same procedure and also made a correction to take into account the reduction in the thickness of the cortex. The most significant results were obtained in young patients, when the reduction in the thickness of the cortex was taken into account. None of these authors also took into account the reduction of the length of the cortical ribbon. If we accept that this is the major factor of atrophy, their results deal mainly with neuronal density, and the pertinence of the results as concerns the real neuronal loss can be discussed.

Cell body density reduction more markedly involves certain neuronal classes, namely middle-sized pyramidal cells. Although this finding has probably been overestimated on account of neuronal atrophy, it is not a mere morphometric artifact (Duyckaerts et al. 1989 b). It suggests, if we accept the columnar hypothesis for atrophy, that the first degenerating cells belong to the pyramidal layers and that columnar atrophy follows.

Senile Changes

The distribution of the main lesions of AD, various types of senile plaques (SP) and neurofibrillary tangles (NFT) has been described by many groups of investigators. The semiquantitative estimation of the severity of both changes and of gliosis and spongiosis in the neocortex done by Brun and Englund (1981) fits well the distribution of the reduction in glucose consumption during AD. However, things are not so clear, since some changes are found in deep structures. Moreover, the distributions of the cortical lesions seen in AD are different according to their types – tangles or different varieties of plaques. Results from different authors are not easy to compare as the same specimen submitted to various staining techniques reveals different densities of lesions (Duyckaerts et al. submitted; Lamy et al. 1989; Wisnieswki et al. 1989b). In addition, densities of individual lesions do not vary at the same rate as a function of the duration of the disease, as seen in the Charles Foix longitudinal study (in preparation). Mann et al. (1988) compared the data of cerebral biopsies to the changes seen at autopsy in the same patients affected with AD. In all five cases, the density and the nucleolar volume of neocortical pyramidal cells fell significantly from biopsy to death. By contrast, in none of the five cases did SP density consistently change. NFT density either did not change or, indeed, sometimes decreased from biopsy to death.

Neurofibrillary Tangles

As far as neurofibrillary tangles are concerned, it is clear that a large preponderance of the changes are in the hippocampus and adjacent areas and in the amyg-

Table 3. Topography of neurofibrillary tangles in aging and in AD[a]

	Normal aging[b]	AD
Hippocampal formation	+	+ + +
Pyramidal cells of the subiculum, CA 1, end plate, etc.		
+Layers II and IV of entorhinal cortex of the parahippocampal gyrus	+ +	+ + +
Amygdala	+	+ + +
Lateral and basal accessory nuclei		
Olfactory bulb	±	+ +
Cortex (other areas)	±	+ +
Pyramidal cells of layers III and V		
Prefrontal > cingular and other association areas > primary areas		
Basal ganglia	±	+ +
Basal magnocellular complex (including nucleus basalis of Meynert), thalamic intralaminar nuclei, lateral hypothalamus and dorsomedial nucleus, etc.		
Brainstem	±	+
Locus ceruleus, dorsal and median raphe nuclei, ventral tegmental area, pedunculopontine and laterodorsal tegmental nuclei, substantia nigra, etc.		
Sympathetic ganglia		

[a] Data from: Ball and Lo (1977), Braak and Braak (1989 a,b), Brun and Englund (1981), Doebler et al. (1987), Duyckaerts et al. (1987), Hansen et al. (1988), Hauw et al. (1986), Herzog and Kemper (1980), Kawasaki et al. (1987), Kemper (1984), Mann (1988), Moosy et al. (1989), Morrison et al. (1987), Saper (1988), Terry et al. (1981, 1987), Tomlinson et al. (1968, 1970), Tomlinson and Corsellis (1984), Ulfig and Braak (1989), Wakabayashi et al. (1989), Wisniewski et al. (1989), Zubenko et al. (1989)
[b] Symbols: ±, scanty or controversial lesions; +, mild lesions; + +, definite lesions; + + +, severe lesions. For AD, crosses indicate lesions more severe than those seen in age-matched controls

Table 4. Topography of SP in aging and in AD[a]

	Normal aging[b]	AD
Hippocampal formation Subiculum, CA1 > CA3, fibrous layers, dentate gyrus molecular layer	+ +	+ + +
Entorhinal cortex of the parahippocampal gyrus	+ +	+ + +
Amygdala Basal magnocellular and basal accessory nuclei	+ +	+ + +
Olfactory bulb	±	+ +
Cortex (other areas) Layers II and III Distribution very diffuse especially in cingular and association areas	+	+ + +
Basal ganglia Basal magnocellular complex, including nucleus of Meynert, > posterolateral and anteroventral thalamic nuclei, lateral hypothalamus, mammillary bodies, etc.	±	+ +
Brainstem Periaqueductal gray, superior colliculus, IVth ventricle floor, reticular formation especially superior central nucleus, substantia nigra, etc.	±	±

[a] Data from: Ball and Lo (1977), Braak and Braak (1989a,b), Brun and Englund (1981), Duyckaerts et al. (1986), Hansen et al. (1988), Hauw et al. (1986), Herzog and Kemper (1980), Iseki et al. (1989), Joachim et al. (1989b), Kemper (1984), Mann (1988), Masliah et al. (1989), Moosy et al. (1989), Morrison et al. (1987), Saper (1988), Tomlinson et al. (1968, 1970), Tomlinson and Corsellis (1984), Wakabayashi et al. (1989), Yamaguchi et al. (1989), Zubenko et al. (1989)

[b] Symbols: ±, scanty or controversial lesions; +, mild lesions; + +, definite lesions; + + +, severe lesions. For AD, crosses indicate lesions more severe than those seen in age-matched controls

dala (Table 3). The subcortical nuclei which are affected usually (or always for some authors) appear to be those which project to the cortex. In the neocortex, tangles most appear in some specific areas, namely association cortices. This is best demonstrated in the occipital cortex, where they spare area 17 and are more and more numerous in areas 18 and 19 (Braak and Braak 1989a).

Senile Plaques

The preponderance of SP also occurs in the hippocampus and adjacent areas and in the amygdala (Table 4). By contrast, SP at least of the mature or classical type, are rarer in most subcortical structures. In the neocortex, they are more numerous than the NFT (Zubenko et al. 1989) and more diffusely spread, as seen in the Charles Foix longitudinal study (in preparation). In addition, recent data obtained with very sensitive techniques (overall immunocytochemistry of β-amyloid and precursors, tau and Alz-50) have enlarged the spectrum of the brain areas involved in the disease; immature SP or other preamyloid deposits have been seen in areas where no (or very few) lesions were seen with conventional techniques, such as the cerebellum or the striatum, to deal only with the brain (Braak and Braak 1989 b; Joachim et al. 1989 a, b; Ulfig and Braak 1989; Wisnieswki et al. 1989 a; Yamaguchi et al. 1989).

Other Changes

The other changes seen in AD sometimes affect the same areas, but sometimes different ones (Table 5). As an example, amyloid angiopathy is more common in the occipital lobe.

Asymmetry of Changes

Although AD is usually described as a disease associated with diffuse atrophy of the cerebral cortex and symmetrical distribution of morphological lesions, their asymmetry in some cases was reported long ago (Delay and Brion 1962). Quantitative data on the extent of lateralization of the lesions in two neocortical areas (middle frontal and superior temporal cortices) and in entorhinal cortex and prosubiculum have been reported recently. Morphologic lesions were more asymmetrically distributed than deficits in cholinergic enzymes, choline acetyltransferase and acetylcholinesterase. Although there were some cases with ratios of left-right asymmetry of up to 9 for SP and 7 for NFT (in mildly affected cases), asymmetries of these lesions did not tend to colateralize (Moosy et al. 1989).

Table 5. Topography of other lesions in AD[a]

Lesion	Topography	Intensity[a]
Abnormal network of fibers and neuropil threads	Hippocampus and neocortex	+ + +
Granulovacuolar degeneration	Hippocampus	+ + +
Hirano bodies	Hippocampus	+ +
Amyloid angiopathy	Occipital cortex	+ + +
	Temporal cortex	+ +
	Other neocortical areas	+
	Cerebellum	±
Diffuse senile plaques and other amyloid deposits (A 4)	Striatum	+ +
	Cerebellum	+
	Cerebral cortex (subpial)	+
	Basal ganglia, white matter, etc.	+
	Skin, etc.	+
PHF, Tau, Alz 50 immunochemistry	Olfactory epithelium	+

[a] Data from: Ball and Lo (1977), Braak et al. (1986), Duyckaerts et al. (1989a), Hansen et al. (1988), Hauw et al. (1986), Joachim et al. (1989a, b), Kemper (1984), Mann (1988), Masliah et al. (1989), Saper (1988), Talamo et al. (1989), Tomlinson et al. (1968, 1970), Tomlinson and Corsellis (1984), Wisniewski et al. (1989a)
[b] Symbols: ±, scanty or controversial lesions; +, mild lesions; + +, definite lesions; + + +, severe lesions. For AD, crosses indicate lesions more severe than those seen in age-matched controls

In conclusion, concerning the distribution of lesions, it can be said that no precise detailed study of the whole range of AD changes in the same prospectively assessed patients is available today. Such as study should take into account gross as well as microscopic findings and should deal with conventional as well as more modern techniques such as immunocytochemistry (Delaère et al. 1989 a,b; Duyckaerts et al. 1988 and submitted; Wisnieswki et al. 1989 a). It could use mental deterioration and other clinical signs as a reference. Validating clinical data by pathology, and pathological data by clinical information, could obviously lead to circular conclusions and should be avoided. However, careful clinicopathological correlation is the only available method to search for the link between lesions and clinical deficits.

Where Do the Changes Begin and How Do They Spread?

If we hypothesize a regular increase of the lesions in each considered area, then we must accept that they begin in the areas where they are the densest. As a matter of fact, this conclusion could be a mirage, since mild changes occurring in large areas could concentrate through anatomical pathways to small structures where they would appear very dense and could be taken as more precocious.

There is no consensus concerning the causes of the distribution of changes in AD. The main hypothetical pathways are: olfactory, "limbic" (Hyman et al. 1984, 1988), associative "corticocortical" (Morrison et al. 1987), corticosubcortical or subcorticocortical. Other explanations for the distribution of lesions in aging and AD have been suggested; the selective vulnerability of some neuronal groups is a well-known feature in neuropathology. Among the suggested explanations are the special metabolism or vascularization of some areas or of specific cell types; the selective involvement of a specific system of neuromediators, possibly through an excitotoxic mechanism; the high sensitivity of long axons related to axonal flow disturbances (Gajdusek 1985), the regional variations of amyloidogenesis or of cerebral blood vessel permeability (which could be due to a loss of cholinergic or monoaminergic influences) and the vulnerability of phylogenetically recent areas (Rapoport 1988). All of these explantions are open to discussion (Mann 1988; Hauw et al. 1989).

Conclusions

There is a striking contrast between some very precisely studied structures (generally small, well-defined nuclei) and other areas which offer resistance to morphologists. These latter areas are often very important structures for neuroimaging purposes. Present data concerning the lesions of the cerebral neocortex and of the hemispheric white matter in AD, and even more in the late-onset forms of the disease, and their distinction from the features of normal aging are still conflicting. This is due to the complexity of the organization of these areas, to the lack of animal models for AD, and to the length and difficulties of prospective studies in a long-lasting disease. Two main strategies have been followed for the study of these changes. A pragmatic "gaussian" one has looked for normative data of aging brain using horizontal studies of whole elderly populations, regardless of their clinical status and risk factors. A more "genetic" one has, more recently tried to set up these data among highly selected, prospectively followed, normal individuals or AD patients. We believe that the clues for understanding the mechanism and topography of changes in aging and AD can only be found using these latter types of study. Neuropathologists still have some work ahead of them.

Acknowledgments. The authors wish to thank Drs. Laforestrie, Poulain and Rainsard (Etude longitudinale Charles Foix) and N. Provost and P. Mielle for their skillful assistance. This work was initiated with the help of INSERM (PRC Santé Mentale et Cerveau – 82:966).

References

Ball MJ, Lo R (1977) Neuronal loss, neurofibrillary tangles and granulovacuolar degeneration in the hippocampus with ageing brain and senile dementia. Acta Neuropathol (Berlin) 37:111–118

Berg L, Danziger WL, Storandt M, Cobern LA, Gado M, Knesevich JW, Botwinick J (1984) Predictive features in mild senile dementia of the Alzheimer type. Neurology 34:563–569

Blanks JC, Blanks HI (1988) Retinal defects in Alzheimer's patients. In: Proceedings of the international symposium on Alzheimer's disease. Kuopio. June 12–15, p 133

Blessed G, Tomlinson BE, Roth M (1968) The association between quantitative measures of dementia and of senile changes in the cerebral gray matter of elderly subjects. Br J Psychiatr 114:797–811

Braak H, Braak E (1989a) Alzheimer's disease: distribution pattern of amyloid and neurofibrillary changes in the occipital cortex. Am Assoc Neuropathol 65th Ann Meet, Abstract 151

Braak H, Braak E (1989b) Amyloid deposits and neurofibrillary changes in the striatum in cases of Alzheimer's disease. Clin Neuropathol 8:222

Braak H, Braak E, Grundke-Iqbal I, Iqbal K (1986) Occurrence of neuropil threads in the senile human brain in Alzheimer's disease. Neurosci Lett 65:351–355

Brun A, Englund E (1981) Regional pattern of degeneration of Alzheimer's disease: neuronal loss and histopathology grading. Histopathology 5:549–564

Brun A, Englund E (1986) A white matter disorder of dementia of the Alzheimer type: a pathoanatomical study. Ann Neurol 19:253–262

Dam AM (1979) The density of neurons in the human hippocampus. Neuropathol Appl Neurobiol 5:249–264

Davis PJM, Wright EA (1977) A new method for measuring cranial capacity volume and its application to the assessment of cerebral atrophy at autopsy. Neuropathol Appl Neurobiol 3:341–358

Dekaban AS, Sadowsky D (1978) Changes in brain weight during the span of human life: relation of brain weight to body height and body weight. Ann Neurol 4:345–356

De la Monte S (1989) Quantification of cerebral atrophy in preclinical and end-stage Alzheimer's disease. Ann Neurol 25:450–459

Delaère P, Duyckaerts C, Brion J-P, Poulain V, Hauw J-J (1989a) Tau, PHF and amyloid in the neocortex: a morphometric study of 15 cases with graded intellectual status in aging and SDAT. Acta Neuropathol (Berl) 77:645–653

Delaère P, Duyckaerts C, Brion J-P, Piette F, Hauw J-J (1989b) Relationship between tau, PHF, amyloid and the intellectual status in aging and senile dementia of Alzheimer type. In: Boller

F, Katzman R, Rascol A, Signoret JL, Christen Y (eds) Biological markers of Alzheimer's disease. Springer, Berlin Heidelberg New York, pp 73–82

Delay J, Brion S (1962) Les démences tardives. Masson, Paris

Doebler JA, Markesberry WD, Anthony A, Rhoads R (1987) Neuronal RNA in relation to neuronal loss and neurofibrillary pathology in the hippocampus in Alzheimer's disease. J Neuropathol Exp Neurol 46:28–39

Duyckaerts C, Brion J-P, Hauw J-J, Flament-Durand J (1987) Quantitative assessment of the density of neurofibrillary tangles and senile plaques in senile dementia of the Alzheimer type. Comparison of immunocytochemistry with a specific antibody and Bodian's protargol method. Acta Neuropathol (Berl) 73:167–170

Duyckaerts C, Delaère P, Poulain V, Brion J-P, Hauw J-J (1988) Does amyloid precede paired helical filaments in the senile plaque? A study of 15 cases with graded intellectual status in aging and Alzheimer disease. Neurosci Letters 91:354–359

Duyckaerts C, Hauw J-J, Bastenaire F, Piette F, Poulain V, Rainsard C, Javoy-Agid F, Berthaux P (1986) Laminar distribution of neocortical senile plaques in senile dementia of the Alzheimer type. Acta Neuropathol (Berl) 70:249–256

Duyckaerts C, Hauw J-J, Piette F, Rainsard C, Poulain V, Berthaux P, Escourolle R (1985) Cortical atrophy in senile dementia of the Alzheimer type is mainly due to a decrease in cortical length. Acta Neuropathol (Berl) 66:72–74

Duyckaerts C, Kawasaki H, Delaère P, Rainsard C, Hauw J-J (1989a) Fiber disorganisation in the neocortex of patients with senile dementia of the Alzheimer type. Neuropathol Appl Neurobiol 15:233–247

Duyckaerts C, Llamas E, Delaère P, Mièle P, Hauw J-J (1989b) Neuronal loss and neuronal atrophy. Computer simulation in connection with Alzheimer's disease. Brain Res, in press

Galen RS, Gambino SR (1975) Beyond normality: the predictive value and efficiency of medical diagnoses. Wiley, New York

Gajdusek DC (1985) Hypothesis: interference with axonal transport of neurofilaments as common mechanism in certain diseases of the central nervous system. New Engl J Med 312:714–719

Hansen LA, De Teresa R, Davies P, Terry R (1988) Neocortical morphometry, lesion counts, and choline acetyltransferase levels in the age spectrum of Alzheimer's disease. Neurology 38:48–54

Haug H, Kühl S, Mecke E, Sass NL, Wasnerk K (1984) The significance of morphometric procedures in the investigation of age changes in cytoarchitectonic structures of human brain. J Hirnforsch 25:353–374

Hauw J-J, Duyckaerts C, Delaère P (1988) Neuropathology of aging and SDAT: how can age-related changes be distinguished from those due to disease process? In: Henderson AS, Henderson JH (eds) Etiology of dementia of Alzheimer type. Dahlem Konferenzen. London, pp 195–211

Hauw J-J, Duyckaerts C, Delaère P (1988) Neuropathology of aging and SDAT. In: Duckett S (ed) The pathology of the aging human brain. Lea and Febiger, Philadelphia, in press

Hauw J-J, Duyckaerts C, Partridge M (1987) Neuropathological aspects of brain aging and SDAT. In: Courtois C, Faucheux B, Forette B, Knook DL, Tréton JA (eds) Modern trends in aging research. Libbey, London, pp 435–442

Hauw J-J, Vignolo P, Duyckaerts C, Beck H, Forette F, Henry J-F, Laurent M, Piette F, Sachet A, Bethaux P (1986) Etude neuropathologique de 12 centenaires. La fréquence de la démence sénile de type Alzheimer n'est pas particulièrement élevée dans ce groupe de personnes très agées. Rev Neurol (Paris) 142:107–115

Herzog AG, Kemper TL (1980) Amygdaloid changes in aging and dementia. Arch Neurol 37:625–629

Hubbard BM, Anderson JM (1981) A quantitative study of cerebral atrophy in old age and senile dementia. J Neurol Sci 50:135–145

Hyman BT, DamasioAR, Van Hoesen GW (1988) Memory-related neural systems are disrupted at multiple levels by Alzheimer's disease. In: Proceed Internat Symp Alzheimer's disease, Kuopio, pp 26–29

Hyman BT, Damasio AR, Van Hoesen GW, Barnes CL (1984) Alzheimer's disease: cell specific pathology isolates the hippocampal formation. Science 225:1168–1170

Iseki E, Matsushita M, Kosaka K, Kondo H, Ishii T, Amano N (1989) Distribution and morphology of brain stem plaques in Alzheimer's disease. Acta Neuropathol (Berlin) 78:131–136

Joachim CL, Mori H, Selkoe DJ (1989a) Amyloid β-protein deposition in tissues other than brain in Alzheimer's disease. Nature 341:226–230

Joachim C, Morris J, Platt D, Selkoe D (1989b) Diffuse senile plaques: the caudate and putamen as a model. Am Assoc Neuropathol. 65th Ann Meet, Abstract 87

Katzman R, Lasker B, Berstein N (1988) Advances in the diagnosis of dementia: accuracy of diagnosis and consequences of misdiagnosis of disorders causing dementia. In: Terry RD (ed) Aging and the brain. Raven, New York, pp 17–62

Kawasaki H, Murayama S, Tomonaga M, Izumiyama N, Shimada H (1987) Neurofibrillary tangles in human upper cervical ganglia; morphological study with immunohistochemistry and electron microscopy. Acta Neuropathol (Berlin) 75:156–159

Kemper T (1984) Neuroanatomical and neuropathological changes in normal aging and in dementia. In: Albert LM (ed) Clinical neurology of aging. Oxford University Press, New York, pp 9–52

Lamy C, Duyckaerts C, Delaère P, Payan Ch, Fermanian J, Poulain V, Hauw J-J (1989) Comparison of seven staining methods for senile plaques and neurofibrillary tangles in a prospective series of 15 elderly patients. Neuropathol Appl Neurobiol 15:in press

Mann DMA (1988) Neuropathology and neurochemical aspects of Alzheimer's disease. In. Iversen LL, Iversen SD, Snyder SH (eds) Psychopharmacology of the aging nervous system. Handbook of psychopharmacology, Vol 20. Plenum, New York, pp 1–67

Mann DMA, Marcyniuk B, Yates PO, Neary D, Snowden JS (1988) The progression of the pathological changes of Alzheimer's disease in frontal and temporal neocortex examined both at biopsy and at autopsy. Neuropathol Appl Neurobiol 14:177–195

Mann DMA, Yates PO, Marcyniuk B (1985) Some morphometric observations on the cerebral cortex and hippocampus in presenile Alzheimer's disease, senile dementia of Alzheimer type and Down syndrome in middle age. J Neurol Sci 69:139–159

Masliah E, Terry R, Buzsahi G (1989) Thalamic nuclei in Alzheimer disease: evidence against the cholinergic hypothesis of plaque formation. Brain Res 493:240–246

Meyer-Ruge W, Ulrich J, Abdel-Al S (1984) Stereologic findings in normal brain aging and Alzheimer's disease. In: Wertheimer J, Marois M (eds) Senile dementia: outlook for the future. Liss, New York, pp 125–135

Miller AKH, Alston RL, Corsellis JAN (1980) Variations with age in the volumes of gray and white matter in the cerebral hemispheres of man: measurements with an image analyser. Neuropathol Appl Neurobiol 6:119–132

Miller AKH, Corsellis JAN (1977) Evidence for a secular increase in human brain weight during the past century. Ann Human Biol 4:253–257

Mountjoy CQ, Roth M, Evans NJR, Evans HM (1983) Cortical neuronal counts in normal elderly controls and demented patients. Neurobiol Aging 4:1–11

Moosy J, Zubenko GS, Martinez AJ, Rao GR, Kopp U, Hanin I (1989) Lateralization of morphologic and cholinergic abnormalities in Alzheimer's disease. Arch Neurol 46:639–642

Morrison JH, Lewis DA, Campbell MJ (1987) Distributions of neurofibrillary tangles and nonphosphorylated neurofilament protein. Immunoreactive neurons in cerebral cortex: implications for loss of corticocortical circuits in Alzheimer's disease. In: Davies P, Finch CE (eds) Molecular neuropathology of aging. Banbury Report 27. Cold Spring Harbor Laboratory, New York, pp 109–124

Rakic P (1988) Specification of cerebral cortical areas. Science 241:170–176

Rapoport SI (1988) Brain evolution and Alzheimer's disease. Rev Neurol (Paris) 144:79–90

Saper CF (1988) Chemical neuroanatomy of Alzheimer's disease. In: Iversen LL, Iversen SD, Snyder SH (eds) Psychopharmacology of the aging nervous system, Handbook of psychopharmacology. Vol 20. Plenum Press, New York, pp 131–156

Sulkava R, Haltia M, Paetau A, Wikström, Palo J (1983) Accuracy of clinical diagnosis in primary degenerative dementia: correlation with neuropathological findings. J Neurol Neurosurg Psychiatry 46:9–13

Swaab DF, Fliers E, Partiman TS (1985) The suprachiasmatic nucleus of the human brain in relation to sex, age and senile dementia. Brain Res 342:37–44

Talamo B, Rudel RA, Kosik KS, Lee V, Neff S, Adelman L, Kauer JS (1989) Pathological changes in olfactory neurons in patients with Alzheimer's disease. Nature 337:736–739

Terry RD, de Teresa R, Hansen LA (1987) Neocortical cell counts in normal human adult ageing. Ann Neurol 21:530–539

Terry RD, Peck A, de Teresa R, Schechter R, Horoupian DS (1981) Some morphometric aspects of the brain in senile dementia of the Alzheimer type. Ann Neurol 10:184–192

Tierney MC, Fisher RH, Lewis AJ, Zorzitto ML, Snow WG, Reid DW, Nieuwstraten P (1988) The NINCDS-ADRDA work group criteria for the clinical diagnosis of probable Alzheimer's disease: a clinico-pathologic study of 57 cases: Neurology 38:359–564

Tomlinson BE, Blessed G, Roth M (1968) Observations on the brain of non-demented old people. J Neurol Sci 7:331–356

Tomlinson BE, Blessed G, Roth M (1970) Observations on the brain of demented old people. J Neurol Sci 11:207–242

Tomlinson BE, Corsellis JAN (1984) Ageing and the dementias: In. Humes Adams J, Corsellis JAN, Duchen LW (eds) Greenfield's neuropathology, Edward Arnold, London, pp 951–1025

Ulfig N, Braak H (1989) Distribution of Alzheimer – typical changes in the hypothalamus. Clin Neuropathol 8:253

Wakabayashi K, Furuta A, Takahashi H, Ikuta F (1989) Occurrence of neurofibrillary tangles in the celiac ganglia. Acta Neuropathol (Berlin) 78:448

Wisniewski HM, Wen GY, Kim KS (1989) Comparison of four methods on the detection of neuritic plaques. Acta Neuropathol (Berlin) 78:22–27

Wisnieswki HM, Bancher C, Barcikowska M, Wen GY, Currie J (1989) Spectrum of morphological appearance of amyloid deposits in Alzheimer's disease. Acta Neuropathol (Berlin) 78:337–347

Yamaguchi H, Hirai S, Morimatsu M, Shoji M, Nakazato Y (1989) Diffuse type of senile plaques in the cerebellum of Alzheimer-type dementia demonstrated by β protein immunostain. Acta Neuropathol 77:314–319

Zubenko GS, Moosy J, Martinez AJ, Rao GR, Kopp U, Hanin I (1989) A brain regional analysis of morphologic and cholinergic abnormalities in Alzheimer's disease. Arch Neurol 46:634–638

Computer Tomography and Study of the Anatomical Changes in Alzheimer's Disease

H. Creasey, J. Luxenberg, M. Schapiro, J. V. Haxby and S. I. Rapoport

The role of anatomical changes in Alzheimer's disease (AD) can be studied using computer tomography (CT) scanning. By comparing carefully selected and screened subjects to appropriately age- and sex-matched healthy controls, atrophy in AD can be shown to be due to excess cortical, but not subcortical, gray matter loss, accompanied by ventricular dilatation and increased total cerebrospinal fluid (CSF) volume. This gray matter loss and increase in CSF volume within the AD group is related to clinical severity at the time of scanning. Although these parameters can distinguish moderate–severe AD cases from controls, much overlap of gray matter volume and of lateral ventricular volume is seen between healthy controls and patients with mild AD (as defined by an MMS score of greater than 20). This is due to the heterogeneity of age-related atrophy seen in healthy controls and patients. Prospective serial scanning and cognitive testing permits study of the rate of change of both atrophy and cognitive functioning within each individual, reducing variability, and show that the rate of change of the third ventricle and lateral ventricular volumes is greater in patients with AD than in healthy controls, separating even mildly affected patients completely from the controls. The rate of atrophy change correlates with the change in global cognitive function, as measured in the AD group by global neuropsychological scores. Asymmetric cognitive decline is reflected in corresponding asymmetric rates of change of lateral ventricular size. Similar results are seen in subjects with Down's syndrome (DS). Older DS subjects developing dementia have accelerated enlargement of lateral ventricular volume in serial CT scans compared to those DS subjects who dot not develop dementia. In nondemented DS subjects, age-related brain atrophy is seen similar to that observed in aging, normal healthy subjects. These studies taken together show that dynamic anatomical changes in AD are an integral part of the disease process and not just end-stage events. Early in the disease, progressive atrophy can be documented and is associated with progressive decline in function. Demonstration of such early progression of atrophy may strengthen a diagnosis of AD and identify subclinical cases. It also has the potential to document changes in atrophy rate in response to therapeutic interventions.

Introduction

Areas of Interest

The advent of CT scanning has made possible macroscopic visual brain images during life. In AD the focus of CT scan studies has been on brain atrophy. Reports of the relationship between CT atrophy and AD have centered on several areas of interest. This paper will focus on five questions in the anatomical study of AD: (1) does the amount of atrophy distinguish patients with AD from controls; (2) does the amount of atrophy relate to the severity of the dementia in AD; (3) does the rate of progression of atrophy distinguish patients with AD from controls; (4) does the rate of progression of atrophy in AD correlate with clinical decline; and (5) in Down's syndrome (DS), is atrophy related to retardation, the premature accumulation of Alzheimer pathology or to clinical dementia. The current understanding of these areas is reviewed here, and studies performed in the Laboratory of Neurosciences (LNS) of the National Institutes on Aging will be presented to illustrate current answers to these questions. Many studies have addressed questions and 2, but the results of these studies have often been conflicting for a variety of reasons. Questions 3 through 5 have been the subjects of only preliminary studies at this stage. The results of such studies, however, are of great interest.

Problems in Methodology

A major problem seen in CT studies of AD, which has led to some of the differing results, is that the methods of measurement have varied widely. Some methods (such as linear measures) poorly reflect the actual amount of atrophy present because they least reflect three-dimensional size, and others (such as ratings) show poor interrater reliability. While linear measures are easy to perform, volumetric measures require computer facilities. These are, however, usually available with the scanner. An example of the difference such measures make is seen in the findings of Gado et al. (1982, 1983), in which volumetric measures show better separation of groups than linear measures, both initially and with serial scanning over a 1-year period. Similar findings have been reported by others (Brinkman et al. 1981; Soininen et al. 1982; Albert et al. 1984). The increase in CSF from brain atrophy can be considered in two components: ventricular and sulcal. An estimate of sulcal fluid volume is usually derived by subtraction of total ventricular volume from total CSF volume and is less accurate than ventricular measures, which are derived directly in most studies. Correspondingly, overall ventricular size measures separate groups more consistently and correlate better with cognitive measures than do sulcal ones.

Variations in head size can influence the size of the ventricles and brain, and linear corrections for head size are often made, although more complex corrections are more accurate.

Computer tomography scanners vary in their image production, and the amount of atrophy seen in the image can vary according to the scanner used. If several different scanners are used, particularly if they differ between patients and controls, artifactual differences may be found or real ones may be missed. The angle of scanning alters the appearance of intracranial structures, and variations in the conditions of the scan (duration of beam, temperature of room, voltage and width of the beam) can alter the image significantly. These can all alter the appearance of the structures to be measured. When viewing scan images, different window settings can alter the apparent amount of atrophy present. Images nearer the vertex are often marred by bone density artifact, which makes direct measurement of sulcal fluid difficult (see above).

Another source of study variability has been definition of patients with dementia and selection of a comparison group where differences from normal have been sought. Some studies have used subjects with dementia regardless of cause, while others have attempted to use patients with probable AD alone. Controls vary from nondemented patient scans to rigorously screened normal volunteers.

Specific Methodology in LNS Studies

In these studies, some of the problems mentioned above have been addressed by using careful selection of patients and controls, using volumetric analyses and a program of standardization of the scanning procedure. Serial clinical assessment has been combined with serial scanning.

Scanning

All scans were obtained on a GE 8800 CT Scanner (General Electric Co, Milwaukee, WI) for which full width at half max (FWHM) equaled 1 mm. Slices were taken 10 mm thick at the center, parallel to and from the inferior orbitomeatal line extending to the vertex. The scanner was standardized daily by an internal standardization program, using a water phantom (CT density = 0 Hounsfield units, HU) and lucite (CT density = 120 HU). CT data were stored on magnetic tape and were displayed on a TV monitor for analysis.

Analysis

A computer-assisted program (DeLeo et al. 1985) permitted categorization of the CT slice into CSF, white matter and gray matter. Samples of CSF, white matter and gray matter were visually identified in a standardized fashion to yield representative ranges of CT densities. The boundaries between CSF and white matter, and between white matter and gray matter, were established. The slice was then analyzed using a nearest-neighbor technique to categorize all pixels in the slice into CSF, white matter or gray matter. The total number of pixels in each category and the percentage relative to the total intracranial pixels in the slice were then derived. Seven consecutive slices, beginning at the slice containing the third ventricle, were used. Higher slices were not analyzed to avoid "beam-hardening" artifact. By summation across the seven slices, and using pixel area ($0.0064\ cm^2$), volumes and volumes as percentages of the seven-slice intracranial segment of each category (CSF, white matter and gray matter) were calculated.

Individual regions within the scan slices were also measured using a region-of-interest program whereby a structure could be outlined on the monitor-displayed scan image using a digitizing tablet, and the number of pixels within the outlined structure could be calculated. Area was calculated from pixel number and pixel size. Summation across slices muliplied by interslice distance permitted calculation of individual structure volumes. Structures studied included the subcortical nuclei (caudate, thalamus and lentiform nuclei), the lateral ventricles (right and left, with their individual frontal and occipital horns) and the third ventricle. Subarachnoid CSF volume was derived only indirectly by subtracting total ventricular volume from the seven-slice total CSF volume.

Interrater reliability was significant for all measures, but higher for the region-of-interest measures than the whole matter volumes. The limited reliability of the latter method reflected the technical limits of CT scanning, in which each pixel is assigned a single whole number value despite, in reality, containing a mixture of tissues of differing density values.

Subject Groups

Patients in the AD group met the DSM-III criteria (American Psychiatric Association 1980) for primary degenerative dementia and the NINCDS-ADRDA criteria (McKhann et al. 1984) for "probable" or "possible" AD. They had no other medical, neurological or psychiatric disease, and underwent standard investigations to exclude other causes of dementia and were medication-free.

The control group was composed of carefully screened healthy normal volunteers who were participants in the NIA LNS Normal Aging Study. They had no history of systemic illness, psychiatric disorder, alcohol or drug abuse and had normal physical examinations and laboratory evaluations. All had at least 12 years of education and none was on medications.

For the DS group, all subjects were living in the community and had trisomy 21 karyotype. All underwent the screening procedures of the AD and healthy controls. Abnormalities that were found included: hypothyroidism, functional systolic murmurs, cataract, B12 deficiency and gait disorder. These disorders were treated where appropriate and none was considered significant in relation to the cognitive functioning of the subject or the extent of brain atrophy found.

Cognitive Testing

Cognitive dysfunction in the AD group was evaluated by the Mini-mental State (MMS; Folstein et al. 1975) Blessed Memory, Information and Concentration

Test and Dementia Scale (BMICT and BDS; Blessed et al. 1968). A subgroup of patients was administered the Wechsler Adult Intelligence Scale (WAIS) and Mattis Dementia Scale (Coblenz et al. 1973). For the cross-sectional study (see below) male patients were divided into three groups based on the Mini-mental State score: mild, >19; moderate, $10-19$; severe <10 (Creasey et al. 1986).

For the longitudinal study (see below), male AD patients were divided into two subgroups: mild (MMS score greater than 20) and moderate–severe (MMS score less than 21) (Luxenberg et al. 1987). In addition, a global cognitive decline score (Grady et al. 1985) was derived using results from an extensive battery of neuropsychological tests administered serially to each patient. This neuropsychological score is sensitive to the varying discrete neuropsychological functional changes which are seen particularly early in the disease.

For DS subjects, a different battery was used, reflecting the underlying cognitive impairment present in all these patients. This battery included measures of general intelligence (the Peabody picture vocabulary test-revised), visuospatial ability (three tests), attention (three tests) and visual recognition memory (one test).

Healthy controls also underwent extensive neuropsychological testing including standard psychometric tests such as the WAIS, Benton Visual Retention Test and Luria test battery. These results are not considered further in this paper.

Atrophy: Patients and Controls

The first question of interest was whether atrophy is a diagnostic indicator of AD. One of the major sources of erroneous diagnosis of dementia shortly after the introduction of CT scanning was the use of the presence of atrophy on CT to make such a diagnosis (Huckman et al. 1975). The reason for such errors is the association between age and atrophy, and the results of studies attempting to distinguish normal elderly from those with dementia have been conflicting. Some authors have not found differences between demented subjects and controls on some measures (Gado and Hughes 1978; Kohlmeyer and Shamena 1980; Brinkman et al. 1981; Soininen et al. 1982; Albert et al. 1984) while others have found significant group differences but with much overlap on a variety of measures (Kohlmeyer and Shamena 1980; Brinkman et al. 1981; Soininen et al. 1982; Gado et al. 1983; Albert et al. 1984; Drayer et al. 1985). Misclassification rates have varied from 5% to 38%.

The failure to clearly differentiate patients from controls has been largely due to this confounding effect of age (Brinkman et al. 1981; Gado et al. 1982; Soininen et al. 1982). Quantitative measures of atrophy, such as ventricular size, show significant increases in size with age. For example, in the LNS of the National Institute on Aging (Schwartz et al. 1985), it has been shown that, even in carefully selected healthy adult men of above-average intelligence, this decline in brain size occurs and is predominantly due to loss of cortical and subcortical gray matter, unaccompanied by cognitive decline but accompanied by increased volume of subarachnoid CSF and of the third and lateral ventricles. The variance of atrophy measures also is increased in the fit old subjects compared to that seen in fit young subjects, with some older subjects showing little atrophy and others a great deal.

The amount of atrophy and the age at which it appears have been variously reported with Zatz et al. (1982) reporting changes only after 60 and Takeda and Matsuzawa (1984) finding linear change throughout adult life. The former study used partially screened volunteers while the latter used non-neurologically diagnosed patients. In the carefully selected males in our study, although age-related changes were seen across adult life, these appeared to be greater after age 60, with a suggestion of an exponential increase thereafter.

Other studies have shown some sex dependency of ventricular size and the age-related rate of atrophy (Hatazawa et al. 1982). This heterogeneity with age contributes to the difficulty of separating healthy age-associated atrophy from that due to AD. Even though the age effects are greatest in those over 60, CT measures of atrophy do not completely separate younger AD subjects from normal subjects (Drayer et al. 1985). It would seem desirable to use age and sex matching when studying AD patients compared to controls.

For our cross-sectional study (Creasey et al. 1986) comparing AD subjects to controls, 30 men (44–85 years, mean, 64.1 years) and 6 women (55–76 years, mean, 63.3 years) were used as controls. Within controls in our study group, CT variables showed significant sex differences even with linear ratios correcting for head size; men were found to have greater CSF and ventricular size than females, even as a percentage of the intracranial space. In the AD group, 22 men and 17 women were used. The age range was 45–84 years for the men (mean, 65.4 years) and 55–81 years for the women (mean, 68.8 years).

Patients and age- and sex-matched controls were compared with each other to see if the gray matter and CSF in the CT scan image of those with AD were different from those of the age-matched controls. Differences in mean values were compared with one-way ANOVA and Student's t statistics with Bonferroni corrections for multiple comparisons. All statistical comparisons were performed using SAS programs (SAS Users Guide 1985). Some of the results are shown in Table 1.

The patients with AD had more brain atrophy and ventricular dilatation than the respective age- and sex-matched controls. While the male AD patients as a group had larger third ventricles and less gray matter than controls, when the group was divided into mild, moderate and severe on the basis of the MMS scores, the male patients with mild AD only differed from the male controls in the size of the third ventricle. The male patients with moderate AD showed increased gray matter loss over controls, and the severe AD males had larger ventricles, more CSF and less cortical gray matter than the controls. The subcortical nuclear volumes were not different between the groups, suggesting that the excess gray matter loss in the AD group was cortical. The female AD patiens showed differences from female controls similar to those seen between the severely affected male AD group and the male controls. The female AD patients were more severely affected as a group than the male AD patients.

Thus even with control for age and sex differences, much overlap was seen in the cross-sectional study between patients with AD and controls. While the third ventricle was larger in the patients than in the controls, there was some overlap

Table 1. Comparisons between patients with AD and age- and sex-matched healthy controls on volumetric CT measures of atrophy

	Controls		AD group			
	Males	Females	Male			Female
			Mild	Moderate	Severe	
n	22	6	10	7	5	17
Percentage ratio of seven-slice volume (%):						
CSF	2.4 ± 0.5	6.3 ± 0.6	5.8 ± 0.7	7.5 ± 1.1	13.3 ± 2.6[a]	10.0 ± 0.9[b]
Gray matter	50 ± 1	53 ± 2	50 ± 1	45 ± 2[a]	41 ± 3[a]	43 ± 1[b]
Ventricles	5.1 ± 0.5	2.2 ± 0.3[c]	5.0 ± 0.6	5.5 ± 0.7	8.4 ± 1.1[a]	7.6 ± 0.7[b]
Ventricular volume (ml):						
Right lateral	19.6 ± 2.0	7.2 ± 1.0[c]	19.2 ± 2.2	19.0 ± 2.5	29.0 ± 4.1[a]	25.0 ± 2.4[b]
Left lateral	21.3 ± 2.4	7.3 ± 1.2[c]	18.4 ± 2.8	23.5 ± 3.4	34.1 ± 3.9[a]	27.8 ± 2.9[b]
III	1.7 ± 0.1	1.0 ± 0.2[c]	2.4 ± 0.2[c]	2.7 ± 0.3[a]	2.5 ± 0.4[a]	2.4 ± 0.2[b]

[a] Male AD: significantly different from male controls
[b] Female AD: significantly different from female controls
[c] Female controls: significantly different from male controls
For all results, $p < 0.05$, using Duncan's multiple range test. All results are mean $\pm$ SE

in the mild males with control values. For lateral ventricular size, overlap was marked in the mild and moderate male AD groups with the controls. This makes use of single scans for diagnostic purposes in any one individual difficult, particularly in early cases where the uncertainty of clinical diagnosis is greatest.

Atrophy: Relationship to Severity of Dementia

The second question of interest in CT and AD was the study of the relationship between the amount of atrophy and the severity of the dementia in patients with AD. Such studies have also produced conflicting results. The study subjects have differed widely in the severity of clinical symptoms and duration of disease and in age and presence of other illnesses. Some studies have studied dementia in general and found either no relationship of cognitive function test scores and measures of CT atrophy (Kaszniak et al. 1979; Jacoby and Levy 1980; Ford and Winter 1981; Soininen et al. 1982; Eslinger et al. 1984) or only weakly positive relationships between some cognitive test scores and some CT measures (Roberts and Caird 1976; Kaszniak et al. 1978; Tsai and Tsuang 1979; Jacoby and Levy 1980; Ford and Winter 1981; Soininen et al. 1982). In studies of AD patients only, variable results have also been found with no relationships being reported by Stefoski et al. (1976); Brinkman et al. (1981), Wilson et al. (1982), George et al. (1983), Albert et al. (1984), and Yerby et al. (1985), and weakly positive relationships reported by Gado and Hughes (1978), Gutzmann and Avdaloff (1980), de

Leon et al. (1981), Arai et al. (1983), Naugle et al. (1985) and Chawluk et al. (1986). Positive studies have often combined normal and demented subjects when correlating amount of CT atrophy to mental test scores, while negative studies have not. Stricter selection of patients and complex analyses deriving composite cognitive function and CT atrophy scores also appear to provide a higher yield of positive results. Overall, ventricular dilatation correlates best with mental status in AD (Merskey et al. 1980; George et al. 1983; Albert et al. 1984).

In the cross-sectional study reported above, within the AD group, the severity of dementia as measured on the scales (MMS, BMICT, BDS and Mattis) correlated significantly with the gray matter loss and increase in CSF. However, correlations between WAIS subtest scores and CT variables were no greater than would be expected by chance. There were more significant correlations with the nonverbal subtests than the verbal ones. However, there was no simple relationship between cognitive function and the degree of atrophy in any one individual. Again this suggests that use of a single scan as a measure of the severity of dementia in a patient is not possible. It is possible that the amount of atrophy in AD is not causal in the clinical symptomatology. However, atrophy is greater in patients than in controls, suggesting that atrophy is related to the clinical presentation.

Atrophy Progression: Patients and Controls

A third question of interest was in serial scanning of patients and controls, which allows for individual rates of change in atrophy to be measured and reduces the "noise" from the heterogeneity seen in age-related atrophy in both patients and controls. Preliminary studies of serial scans show increased rates of enlargement of ventricular size in AD subjects over either controls at 1 year, as measured by a variance ratio of several CT measures (Gado et al. 1983: linear and volumetric measures), or cross-sectional normative data (Brinkman and Largen 1984: rate of change of ventricular/brain ratios). Bird (1986) found a greater increase in rate of change of atrophy in normal subjects who developed dementia at follow-up than in those normal subjects who did not develop dementia. Whether the atrophy rate was related to clinical deterioration was not addressed by any of these studies.

In the LNS longitudinal study (Luxenberg et al. 1987), subjects were prospectively studied using the same scanner. Eighteen patients with AD (12 male) underwent serial scans, with a mean interscan interval of 508 days for the males and 450 days for the females.

Twelve of the male controls were also rescanned at an average interscan interval of 1197 days. These 12 males had equivalent education and were of comparable age to the 12 AD males who underwent serial scanning. Some of the results are shown in Table 2.

The rate of change of ventricular volume was calculated by subtracting the most recent scan volume from the volume on the initial scan, then dividing by the time interval between scans (milliliters/year). Final and initial volumes were compared using paired Student's t tests. ANOVA with Bonferroni corrections was

Table 2. Comparisons for rate of change of atrophy: differences from zero in all groups (patients with AD and controls) and differences between male patients with AD and male controls. (Numbers in parenthesis, number of patients in each group)

	Age	Annual increase in ventricular volume [a]		
		Third	Right lateral	Left lateral
Controls (12)	65.1 ± 4.3	0.27 ± 0.06 [b]	-0.23 ± 0.17	-0.29 ± 0.20
Male AD (12)	62.8 ± 2.3	1.2 ± 0.32 [b, c]	6.61 ± 1.29 [b, c]	6.72 ± 0.98 [b, c]
Mild (8)		0.83 ± 0.25 [b]	6.33 ± 1.59 [b, c]	6.93 ± 1.29 [b, c]
Moderate–severe (4)		1.93 ± 0.73 [b, c, d]	7.15 ± 2.52 [b, c]	6.30 ± 1.64 [b, c]
Female AD (6)	70.8 ± 1.7	0.94 ± 0.21 [b]	6.72 ± 1.80 [b]	5.79 ± 2.34

[a] Measured in ml/year $\pm$ SE
[b] Significantly different from zero ($p < 0.05$)
[c] Significantly different from controls ($p < 0.05$)
[d] Significantly different from mild ($p < 0.05$)

used to compare group means. Only male AD patients were compared to male controls with regard to rate of atrophy.

In the serial scan AD study, the mean initial third ventricular volumes did not differ between the mild AD cases and the controls. The moderate–severe AD cases had larger mean initial third ventricular volumes than either the mild AD cases or the controls. The lateral ventricular volumes did not differ among the groups.

The male controls showed a significant increase in third, but not lateral, ventricular volume on serial scanning. In the male AD patients, the rate of third and lateral ventricular enlargement was greater than zero and greater than in controls. The female AD patients showed a significant increase in third and right lateral ventricular volumes on serial scanning. In comparing the mild AD cases to the moderate–severe cases, the change in lateral ventricular volume was not different, but the third ventricular change was greater in the more demented group. There was no overlap of lateral ventricular rates between patients and controls, even those mildly affected. while the third ventricular volumes did show 25% overlap, which was no greater in the mildly affected group than in the controls.

These findings suggest serial studies can be used to distinguish patients with AD from controls, even where initial measures of atrophy do not differ between the groups. The accelerated atrophy of AD thus differs from that of normal aging.

Atrophy Progression: Relationship to Cognitive Decline

This relationship has not been studied other than in the LNS longitudinal study, which showed that the rate of atrophy is related to cognitive decline. Relations between cognitive scores and CT measures were evaluated using Spearman correlational analysis. Global cognitive decline, as measured by rate of change of a global neuropsychological score, correlated with the rate of third and right lateral ventricular enlargement. Great heterogeneity was seen in the rates. For most patients, there was no asymmetry in the rate of lateral ventricular enlargement. However, for those with the most asymmetry initially (>2 SD of controls), asymmetric progression was seen, with the larger ventricle enlarging significantly more than the smaller. These asymmetric progressions correlated with progressive metabolic abnormalities on positron emission tomography (PET) (Luxenberg 1988).

This result would suggest that atrophy accompanies the clinical progression of AD, implying that most of the brain tissue lost in AD occurs with the clinical symptoms rather than preceding or following the clinical profile. This finding has potential clinical use. For example, demonstration of a slowing in the rate of atrophy could provide and objective tool for the evaluation of any postulated curative therapy and should, therefore, be useful in future therapeutic trials. Where clinical decline exceeds the rate of progression of atrophy, another cause for the decline might be suggested.

Down's Syndrome: Relationship Between Atrophy and Function

The final question of interest for CT and AD discussed in this paper is the study of adults with DS. The phenotype of DS is characterized by dementia in up to 50% of patients over 35 years of age (Zellweger 1977), with the neuropathology of the dementia being indistinguishable from that seen in AD (Wisniewski et al. 1985; Mann et al. 1984; Yates et al. 1983; Ball and Nuttal 1981). Whether this neuropathology of DS is accompanied by the same progressive cortical atrophy as seen in AD sufferers who do not have DS has not been explored previously. The question of whether the brain morphology in DS subjects who are demented differs from that found in those DS adults over 45 years who suffer from mental retardation alone was also addressed.

In a cross-sectional study 18 young adult DS subjects (12 male, ages 19–34 years) and 7 older DS subjects (6 male, ages 37–63 years) were compared to 16 young normal males (21–35 years) and 26 middle-aged normal males (36–66 years). One old DS subject was demented (63-year-old male). Quantitative CT showed that young adults with trisomy 21 have small brains, reflecting their small stature and smaller cranial vaults (Schapiro et al. 1985; 1987b). The mental retardation of the young DS adult was not related to cerebral atrophy. While there were no differences between nondemented older and younger adult DS groups in volume of CSF, gray + white matter, or ventricle size, either directly or after normalizing to seven-slice volume, CSF and ventricular volume increased with age, with the same regression slope as found in the healthy controls with age, indicating that the rate of brain atrophy with aging in DS is not different from that in healthy subjects. There were no differences between young and old DS subjects in total intracranial volume or seven-slice volume, as was similarly found in the healthy normal group between young and old subjects.

In a second study, 12 young DS adults (21–33 years, nine males, mean age 25.3 years), five older nondemented DS adults (45–63 years, four males, mean age 52.3 years) and three older demented DS subjects (a 63-year-old male and females aged 55 and 51 years) were scanned allowing comparison of demented and nondemented DS subjects. The demented DS subjects had significantly larger CSF and third ventricular volumes, both absolutely and relative to seven-slice volume, than the younger DS subjects and the nondemented older subjects. The total ventricular volume was increased in demented compared to young and nondemented older DS subjects, respectively. There was no significant difference in ventricular asymmetry among the groups.

Serial scanning was also undertaken for this group of DS subjects (Schapiro et al. 1987a; Schapiro, 1988). All had two or more scans, separated by an average of 43 months for the young, 20 months for the nondemented older and 22 months for the demented older subjects.

The rate of change of a volume of an intracranial structure in milliliters per year was derived from the slope of the regression equation of that volume (ml) on time (years). The mean rate of enlargement of the third ventricle in the patients with dementia and DS did not differ significantly from mean rates in young patients with DS or from the mean rates in older patients with DS who did not have dementia. The rate of change of CSF volume was slightly increased in the nondemented older DS subjects compared to the young DS subjects. Greater rate of change of CSF volume, and for the right and left lateral ventricular volumes, was noted between young and demented old, and for the CSF volume and right lateral ventricle volume between demented old and nondemented old subjects.

Table 3. Comparison of demented older DS subjects with young adult DS subjects and nondemented older DS subjects on initial CT scan measures and annual change in measures derived from serial scans

Measure of atrophy	DS subject groups		
	Young	Older non demented	Older demented
Third ventricle			
Initial[a]	0.62±0.2	0.66±0.27	2.43±0.4[b, c]
Annual change[d]	−0.027±0.056	0.115±0.232	−0.131±0.599
Right lateral ventricle			
Initial	7.7±5.0	7.2±6.5	14.7±2.3
Annual change	−0.27±0.58	0.00±0.75	3.91±2.14[b, c]
Left lateral ventricle			
Initial	9.9±6.0	8.8±8.3	16.5±4.0
Annual change	−0.52±0.51	0.00±0.76	2.18±2.99[b]
CSF volume			
Initial	25.5±13.4	18.6±14.0	50.9±11.2[b, c]
Annual change	−1.32±1.90	2.50±1.81[b]	10.90±4.32[b, c]

[a] ml, mean ± SD
[b] Different from young DS subjects
[c] Different from nondemented older DS subjects
[d] ml/year, mean ± SD

Thus in DS, adult brains are smaller than normal healthy subjects but are not atrophic. Atrophy does occur with age, but at a rate similar to that of normal healthy aging. With clinical dementia in DS subjects, increased rate of atrophy occurs, as is seen in other clinical AD subjects. Some of these results are shown in Table 3.

Conclusions

The controls used in the studies reported here were very healthy and, therefore, would be expected to highlight differences from normal more than controls selected from random samples of elderly subjects in the general population or from non-neurologic patient groups. However, even with this highly selected group, some atrophy with age was seen in the control subjects. This was also the case in the older nondemented DS group, where there was only slight change with age. In the normal controls, changes in cognitive fucntion with age were present (with significant reduction in WAIS Performance Scale Scores) and in older nondemented DS subjects, cognitive function could also be shown to be reduced compared to younger DS subjects (in areas of language, visuospatial and visual memory function). However, these declines were not related to the amount of atrophy seen in these nondemented groups.

Despite the careful selection of controls, use of volumetric measures and standardization of the procedures, overlap between controls and patients in the cross-sectional studies indicates that the absolute amount of atrophy is less important than the individual's change in the amount of atrophy. This is supported by the serial scan studies.

In dementia, there is a documented acceleration of atrophy and cognitive decline which appear to progress together. In AD this would appear to commence in the third ventricular area and then involve cortical gray matter loss, with a concomitant increase in lateral ventricular size and sulcal size. This pattern of loss of brain tissue has been found by Arai et al. (1983) and by Hubbard and Anderson (1981), with the latter study being in autopsied brains.

The rate of change in atrophy seen in AD can reliably separate patients from controls and, as shown for the first time in these studies, is correlated to cognitive and metabolic changes. The complete separation of AD males from control males on total lateral ventricular volume change could be used as a diagnostic marker in those early cases where clinical decline may be subtle or unapparent.

These findings are supported by blood flow studies using ^{133}Xe (Barclay et al. 1984), where a faster rate of decline in blood flow is seen in AD cases than in controls, and within the AD cases has been shown to differentiate those with behavioral decline from those without such decline.

In DS, accelerated brain atrophy must be present to accompany dementia in older DS subjects. Perhaps the AD process in DS occurs in two stages: (1) a microscopic neuropathological process with little atrophy and with cognitive decline short of dementia (Wisniewski et al. 1985; Haberlund, 1969), and (2) a macroscopic loss of brain tissue with clinical dementia. Other studies have shown that dementia in DS is accompanied by atrophy (Dalton and Crapper 1977; Lott and Lai 1982). It has been postulated that this is related to the accelerated tangle formation which correlates with cell loss (Mann and Esiri 1989; Haberlund 1969; Burger and Vogel 1973) and with fewer hippocampal pyramidal cells at autopsy in those DS subjects who die demented (Ball et al. 1986). CT can help distinguish dementia from lesser cognitive decline in old DS subjects, as the mental retardation is not related to cerebral atrophy. In premorbidly normal individuals, accelerated ventricular dilatation can be demonstrated early and the illness lasts a shorter time than in DS.

These findings of progressive atrophy relating to progression of disease process may well apply to other dementias (Damasio et al. 1983) and may be predictive of the development of dementia in clinically apparently normal subjects (Bird et al. 1986). It also provides a means of detecting changes in the rate of disease progression if some successful therapeutic agent is developed, similar to the reversal of atrophy which has been documented in alcoholics who stop drinking (Artmann et al. 1981).

References

Albert M, Naeser MA, Levine HL, Garvery AJ (1984) Ventricular size in patients with presenile dementia of the Alzheimer's type. Arch Neurol 41:1258–1263

American Psychiatric Association Task Force on Nomenclature and Statistics (1980) Diagnostic and statistical manual of mental disorders 3rd edn. American Psychiatric Association, Washington, pp 124–126

Arai H, Kobayashi K, Ikeda K, Nagao Y, Ogihara R, Kosaka K (1983) A computed tomography study of Alzheimer's disease. J Neurol 229:69–77

Artmann H, Gall MV, Hacker H, Herrlich J (1981) Reversible enlargement of cerebral spinal fluid spaces in chronic alcoholics. AJNR 2:23–27

Ball MJ, Nuttal K (1981) Topography of neurofibrillary tangles and granulovacuoles in hippocampi of patients with Down's syndrome: quantitative comparison with normal ageing and Alzheimer's disease. Neuropathol Appl Neurobiol 7:13–20

Ball MJ, Schapiro MB, Rapoport SI (1986) Neuropathological relationships between Down syndrome and senile dementia Alzheimer type. In: Epstein C (ed) The neurobiology of Down syndrome. Raven, New York, pp 45–58

Barclay L, Zemcov A, Blass JP, McDowell F (1984) Rates of decrease of cerebral blood flow in progressive dementias. Neurology 34:1555–1560

Bird JM, Levy R, Jacoby RJ (1986) Computed tomography in the elderly: changes over time in a normal population. Br J Psychiat 148:80–85

Blessed G, Tomlinson BE, Roth M (1968) The association between quantitative measures of dementia and of senile change in the cerebral gray matter of elderly subjects. Br J Psychiat 114:797–811

Brinkman SD, Sarwar M, Levin HS, Morr HH III (1981) Quantitative indexes of computed tomography in dementia and normal aging. Radiology 138:89–92

Brinkman SD, Largen JW Jr (1984) Changes in brain ventricular size with repeated CAT scans in suspected Alzheimer's disease. Am J Psychiat 141:81–83

Burger PC, Vogel FS (1973) The development of the pathologic changes of Alzheimer's disease and senile dementia in patients with Down's syndrome. Am J Pathol 73:457–476

Chawluk J, Alavi A, Hurtig H, Dann R, Bais S, Zimmerman RA, Reivich M (1986) Cerebral atrophy is highly correlated with the severity of Alzheimer's dementia: a volumetric computed tomographic study. Neurology 36 (Suppl 1):264

Coblentz JM, Mattis S, Zingesser LH, Kasoff SS, Wisniewski HM, Katzman R (1973) Presenile dementia: clinical aspects and evaluation of cerebrospinal fluid dynamics. Arch Neurol 29:299–308

Creasey H, Schwartz M, Frederickson H, Haxby JV, Rapoport SI (1986) Quantitative computed tomography in dementia of the Alzheimer type. Neurology 36:1563–1568

Dalton AJ, Crapper DR (1977) Down's syndrome and aging of the brain. In: Mittler P (ed), Research to practice in mental retardation, Vol 3. University Park Press, Baltimore, pp 391–400

Damasio H, Eslinger P, Damasio AR, Rizzo M, Huang HK, Demeter S (1983) Quantitative computed tomographic analysis in the diagnosis of dementia. Arch Neurol 40:715–719

DeLeo JM, Schwartz M, Creasey H, Cutler N, Rapoport SI (1985) Computer-assisted categorization of brain computerized tomography pixels into cerebrospinal fluid, white matter, and gray matter. Comput Biomed Res 18:79–88

de Leon M, George AE, Ferris SH, Reisberg B, Kricheff I (1981) Computer tomography evaluations of brain–behavior relationships in senile dementia. Int J Neurosci 12:246–247

Drayer BP, Heyman A, Wilkinson W, Barrett L, Weinberg T (1985) Early-onset Alzheimer's disease: an analysis of CT findings. Ann Neurol 17:407–410

Eslinger PJ, Damasio H, Graff-Radford N, Damasio AR (1984) Examining the relationship between computed tomography and neuropsychological measures in normal and demented elderly. J Neurol Neurosurg Psychiat 47:1319–1325

Folstein MF, Folstein SE, McHugh PR (1975) "Mini-mental state" – a practical method for grading the cognitive state of patients for the clinician. J Psychiatr Res 12:189–198

Ford CV, Winter J (1981) Computerized axial tomograms and dementia in elderly patients. J Gerontol 36:164–169

Gado M, Hughes C (1978) Cerebral atrophy and ageing. J Comp Ass Tomogr 2:520–522

Gado M, Hughes CP, Danziger W, Chi D, Jost G, Berg L (1982) Volumetric measurements of the cerebrospinal fluid spaces in demented subjects and controls. Radiology 144:535–538

Gado M, Hughes CP, Danziger W, Chi D (1983) Aging, dementia, and brain atrophy: a longitudinal computed tomographic study. AJNR 4:699–702

George A, de Leon MJ, Rosenbloom S, Ferris SH, Gentes C, Emmerich M, Kricheff II (1983) Ventricular volume and cognitive deficit: a computed tomographic study. Radiology 149:493–498

Grady CL, Haxby J, Sundaram M, Berg G, Rapoport S (1985) Longitudinal relations between cognitive and cerebral metabolic deficits in Alzheimer's disease [Abstract]. J Clin Exp Neuropsychol 7:622

Gutzmann H, Avdaloff W (1980) Mental impairment (dementia) and cerebral atrophy in geriatric patients. Mech Ageing Develop 14:459–468

Haberland C (1969) Alzheimer's disease in Down syndrome: clinical-neuropathological observations. Acta Neurol Belg 69:369–380

Hatazawa J, Ito M, Yamaura H, Matsuzawa T (1982) Sex difference in brain atrophy during aging: a quantitative study with computed tomography. J Am Geriatr Soc 30:235–239

Hubbard BM, Anderson JM (1981) A quantitative study of cerebral atrophy in old age and senile dementia. J Neurol Sci 50:135–145

Huckman MS, Fox J, Topel J (1975) The validity of criteria for the evaluation of cerebral atrophy by computed tomography. Radiology 116:85–92

Jacoby RJ, Levy R (1980) Computed tomography in the elderly. II Senile dementia: diagnosis and functional impairment. Br J Psychiat 136:256–269

Kaszniak AW, Garron DC, Fox JH, Bergen D, Huckman M (1979) Cerebral atrophy, EEG slowing, age, education, and cognitive functioning in suspected dementia. Neurology 29:1273–1279

Kohlmeyer K, Shamena A-R (1980) The size of the lateral ventricles and cortical sulci in old age subjects with and without dementia. Neuroradiology 20:271–272

Lott IT, Lai FL (1982) Dementia in Down syndrome. Ann Neurol 12:120

Luxenberg JS, Haxby JV, Creasey H, Sundaram M, Rapoport SI (1987) Rate of ventricular enlargement in dementia of the Alzheimer type (DAT) correlates with rate of neuropsychological deterioration. Neurology 37:1135–1140

Luxenberg J (1988) Imaging studies of brain anatomy. In: Friedland RP (moderator), Alzheimer's disease: clinical and biological heterogeneity. Ann Intern Med 109:304–305

McKhann G, Drachman D, Folstein M, Katzman R, Price D, Stadlan EM (1984) Clinical diagnosis of Alzheimer's disease: report of the NINCDS-ADRDA work group under the auspices of Department of Health and Human Services Task Force on Alzheimer's disease. Neurology 34:939–944

Mann DMA, Yates PO, Marcyniuk B (1984) Alzheimer's presenile dementia, senile dementia of Alzheimer type and Down's syndrome in middle age form an age related continuum of pathological changes. Neuropathol Appl Neurobiol 10:185–207

Mann DMA, Esiri MM (1989) The pattern of acquisition of plaques and tangles in the brains of patients under 50 years of age with Down's syndrome. J Neurol Sci 89:169–179

Merskey H, Ball MJ, Blume WT, Fox AJ, Fox H, Hersch EL, Kral VA, Palmer RB (1980) Relationships between psychological measurements and cerebral organic changes in Alzheimer's disease. Can J Neurol Sci 7:45–49

Naugle RI, Callum CM, Bigler ED, Massman PJ (1985) Neuropsychological and computerized axial tomography volume characteristics of empirically derived dementia subgroups. J nerv Ment Dis 173:596–604

Roberts MA, Caird FI (1976) Computerised tomography and intellectual impairment in the elderly. J Neurol Neurosurg Psychiatry 39:986–989

SAS User's Guide: Statistics, Version 5 Edition (1985) SAS Institute, Cary, North Carolina

Schapiro MB, Creasey H, Schwartz M, Rapoport SI, Cutler NR (1985) Computed tomography (CT) analysis of brain morphometrics in adult Down's syndrome. Neurology 35 (suppl 1):194

Schapiro MB, Luxenberg J, Kaye J, et al. (1987a) Serial quantitative computed tomography (CT) analysis of brain morphometry in adult Down syndrome at different ages [Abstract]. Ann Neurol 22:432

Schapiro MB, Creasey H, Schwartz M, Haxby JV, White B, Moore A, Rapoport SI (1987b) Quantitative CT analysis of brain morphometry in adult Down's syndrome at different ages. Neurology 37:1424–1427

Schapiro MB (1988) Alzheimer disease in premorbidly normal persons with the Down syndrome: disconnection of neocortical brain regions. In: Friedland RP (moderator), Alzheimer's disease: clinical and biological heterogeneity. Ann Intern Med 109:305–307

Schwartz M, Creasey H, Grady CL, DeLeo JM, Frederickson HA, Cutler NR, Rapoport SI (1985) Computed tomographic analysis of brain morphometrics in 30 healthy men, aged 21 to 81 years. Ann Neurol 17:146–157

Soininen H, Puranen M, Riekkinen PJ (1982) Computed tomography findings in senile dementia and normal aging. J Neurol Neurosurg Psychiat 45:50–54

Stefoski D, Bergen D, Fox J, Morrell F, Huckman M, Ramsey R (1976) Correlation between diffuse EEG abnormalities and cerebral atrophy in senile dementia. J Neurol Neurosurg Psychiat 39:751–755

Takeda S, Matsuzawa T (1984) Brain atrophy during aging: a quantitative study using computed tomography. J Am Geriatr Soc 32:520–524

Tsai L, Tsuang MT (1979) The mini-mental state test and computerised tomography. Am J Psychiat 136:436–439

Wilson RS, Fox JH, Huckman MS, Bacon LD, Lobick JJ (1982) Computed tomography in dementia. Neurology 32:1054–1057

Wisniewski KE, Wisniewski HM, Wen GY (1985) Occurrence of neuropathological changes and dementia of Alzheimer's disease in Down's syndrome. Ann Neurol 17:278–282

Yates CM, Simpson J, Gordon A, et al. (1983) Catecholamines and cholinergic enzymes in pre-senile and senile Alzheimer-type dementia and Down's syndrome. Brain Res 280:119–126

Yerby MS, Sundsten JW, Larson EB, Wu SA, Sumi SM (1985) A new method of measuring brain atrophy: the effect of aging in its application for diagnosing dementia. Neurology 35:1316–1320

Zatz LM, Jernigan TL, Ahumada AJ Jr (1982) Changes on computed cranial tomography with aging: intracranial fluid volume. AJNR 3:1–11

Zellweger H (1977) Down syndrome. In: Vinken PJ, Bruyn GW (eds) Handbook of clinical neurology, vol 31. North Holland, New York, 1977, pp 367–469

Could "Leuko-araïosis" Be Secondary to Wallerian Degeneration in Alzheimer's Disease? *

D. Leys, J-P. Pruvo, M. Parent, P. Vermersch, G. Soetaert, M. Steinling, A. Delacourte, A. Défossez, A. Rapoport, J. Clarisse, and H. Petit

Summary

To determine the possible role of Wallerian degeneration in the pathogenesis of "leuko-araïosis" (LA), we studied brain computer-tomography scans of 98 normotensive and nondiabetic subjects free of cardiac diseases: 32 with Alzheimer's disease (AD), 36 with Parkinson's disease (PD), 8 with progressive supranuclear palsy (PSP), and 22 controls. Our study revealed that: (1) in AD, LA scores were greater than in control subjects; (2) in AD, LA was more prominent in posterior periventricular areas, whereas in PD and PSP, LA was more prominent in anterior periventricular areas; (3) in two patients with AD and LA, autopsy revealed diffuse white matter pallor, limited hyaline thickening of small white matter vessels, and mild fibrillary astrocytosis, without any infarction or hypertensive change; and (4) changes were more severe in white matter close to cortical areas with a great density of neurofibrillary tangles but not to cortical areas with a great density of senile plaques. The high LA scores in AD suggested that a factor of LA might be more severe or more widespread in AD than in PD, PSP and normal aging. Differences in the location of LA between the four groups might be due to differences in the location of the gray matter disorder, and might be explained by a Wallerian degeneration phenomenon rather than senile plaques, neurofibrillary tangles or amyloid angiopathy, which have the same location in AD, PD, PSP and normal aging. In addition to previously reported factors, Wallerian degeneration may be another extracerebral predisposing factor of LA.

Symmetrical periventricular and subcortical white matter lucencies have been reported in healthy elderly subjects, using CT scans (Steingart et al. 1987 a; Rezek et al. 1987). They are correlated to age, mean systolic blood pressure, and previous cardiovascular diseases, but not to sex (Steingart et al. 1987 a; Rezek et al. 1987; Inzitari et al. 1987; Kinkel et al. 1985). In demented patients they are correlated to the severity of the dementia and to the presence of neurological abnormalities (Steingart et al. 1987 b). They are more frequent in multi-infarct dementia than in Alzheimer's disease (AD) (Steingart et al. 1987 b; Gupta et al. 1988; Aharon-Peretz et al. 1988).

* This study was supported by grants from INSERM (grant CAR 489016), University Lille II, and the Société de Médecine du Nord.

In 1987 Hachinski et al. called these periventricular white matter lucencies, whose clinical significance and pathogenesis are not clearly established, "leuko-araïosis" (LA). In hypertensive subjects LA is usually attributed to subcortical vascular changes and the terms "subcortical arteriosclerotic encephalopathy" (Kinkel et al. 1985; Loizou et al. 1981) or "Binswanger's disease" (Aharon-Peretz et al. 1988; De Reuck et al. 1980) are commonly applied. Nevertheless, Rezek et al. (1987) in a study of five patients with LA and definite AD found only diffuse white matter pallor, mild fibrillary astrocytosis and hyaline mural thickening of small cerebral arteries, without any hypertensive vascular change or infarction.

The current study was undertaken to determine the possible role of Wallerian degeneration in the pathogenesis of LA in AD.

Subjects and methods

Subjects

Ninety-eight subjects were included in this study: 32 with AD, 36 with Parkinson's disease (PD), 8 with progressive supranuclear palsy (PSP) and 22 controls. To screen out subjects with risk factors shown to be associated with LA (Steingart et al. 1987a; Rezek et al. 1987; Kinkel et al. 1985; Loizou et al. 1981; De Reuck et al. 1980; Huang et al. 1985) and to compare homogeneous groups differing only by their neurological state (AD, PD, PSP, controls), we only included normotensive and nondiabetic subjects free of cardiac diseases. Hypertension was defined using the rules of Inzitari et al. (1987), as the presence of one or more of the following: (1) a systolic blood pressure greater than 160 mmHg or a diastolic blood pressure greater than 90 mmHg, (2) a previous medical diagnosis of hypertension and (3) previous or current treatment for hypertension. Diabetes mellitus was defined as the presence of one or more of the following: (1) a glucose blood level greater than 1.05 g/l using glucose oxidase technique; (2) a previous medical diagnosis of diabetes mellitus and (3) previous or current treatment using antidiabetic drugs. Cardiac disorder was defined as the presence of any abnormality on clinical examination or electrocardiogram, except a right bundle branch block. None of these 98 subjects had evidence of neurologic disease other than AD, PD or PSP, including toxic, focal cerebrovascular disease, or any metabolic disorder involving the glia. None of them had abnormal motor findings, symptomatic infarctions or small focal lucencies consistent with lacunar infarcts, according to Steingart's criteria (Steingart et al. 1987a and b).

The diagnosis of probable AD was made according to National Institute for Neurologic and Communicative Disorders and Stroke/Alzheimer's Disease and Related Disorder Association criteria (McKhann et al. 1984). The AD group included 20 women and 12 men with a mean age of 65.63 years (range, 51–80 years), and a mean mini-mental state examination (MMSE) score (Folstein et al. 1975) of 11.34 (range, 0–23). None of these patients had myoclonus or extrapyramidal disorder. Twenty-four had early-onset AD (onset before 65) and eight had late-onset AD. None of them had a definite familial history of AD, but 10 patients had 1 parent affected by dementia. These subjects underwent a comprehensive laboratory evaluation consisting of an automated blood chemistry battery and tests for vitamin B_{12} deficiency and thyroid dysfunction. They scored two or less on the modified Hachinski's vascular score (Loeb and Gandolfo 1983). Several patients had previously participated in studies on brain atrophy (Leys et al. 1989a), or single photon emission tomography (Leys et al. 1989b).

The diagnosis of PD was established according to Adams and Victor's standard criteria (1985). The PD group included 23 women and 13 men, with a mean age of 68.17 years (range, 50–81 years) and a mean MMSE score of 25.58 (range, 15–30).

The diagnosis of PSP was established according to Blin's criteria of definite PSP (Blin et al. 1989). This group included five women and three men, with a mean age of 71.75 years (range, 66–83 years) and a mean MMSE score of 20.63 (range, 15–27).

Control subjects were patients aged 50 or older examined consecutively over a period of 5 months. They received brain CT scans a few days before the study for diseases which are known not to modify morphological brain structures. Their CT scans had been performed for secondary symptoms attributed to migraine (eight cases), idiopathic trigeminal neuralgia (two cases), temporal arteritis (two cases), Ménière's syndrome (three cases), spinal neurinoma (one case), long-term sequelae of a bacterial dorsal epiduritis (one case), spinal compression by cervical arthrosis (one case), and Bell's palsy (four cases). We excluded patients with the clinical diagnosis of multiple sclerosis, neoplasm, stroke, trauma, hydrocephalus and neurodegenerative disorders. This group included 15 women and seven men with a mean age of 65.96 (range, 50–87 years) and a MMSE score greater than 27 (mean 29.09; range, 28–30).

Statistical analysis failed to reveal any difference between the four groups of subjects based on sex (Chi-square test) and age (ANOVA one way).

Methods

Computer Tomography Scans

The noncontrast CT scans were performed on CE 12000 (CGR, France) or on Siemens Somatom II (Siemens, FRG) using 10-mm contiguous slice thickness in the Virchov's plane. Scan times were 9.6 s/slice. The scans were interpreted from films using the method of Rezek et al. (1987) for systematic evaluation of LA in 15 areas in each hemisphere, including 14 white matter regions and the basal ganglia-thalamic regions, of 4 CT slices. An area was considered lucent if the density was between that of normal white matter and CSF. Severity of a lucency was scored from 0 (no lucency) to 6 (severe lucency wider than 2 cm^2), according to Rezek's scoring system (1987) based on size (< 2 cm^2, $= 2$ cm^2 or > 2 cm^2) and degree (absent, mild or severe) of contrast difference with surrounding brain.

Lucencies due to artifacts (e.g., partial volume effect) were excluded. Ratings were performed separately by two observers (DL and JPP) without knowledge of diagnoses, ages and MMSE scores. The lucency score was the sum of scores assigned by each observer. A score of 0–360 (2 observers/15 areas/2 hemispheres/ maximum score of 6 by area) was determined for each patient and was called the "LA score." The posterior/anterior assymetry was assessed by the index (LAp-LAa)/LA, in which LAp is the sum of LA scores in posterior areas of both hemispheres, corresponding to the areas d-e-h-i-l-m-o as defined by Rezek et al. (1987) and LAa is the sum of LA scores in anterior areas, corresponding to the areas a-b-f-g-j-k-n of both hemispheres.

Neuropathologic Correlates

We studied the white matter in seven regions using hematoxylin-eosin, Luxol and Bodian staining methods, and by immunohistochemistry with anti-GFAP antibodies (Laboratory Dako). White matter lesions were ranked as mild, moderate or severe, according to Brun and Englund's criteria (1986). In the related cortex, senile plaques (SP) detected by Bodian staining and neurofibrillary tangles (NFT) detected by anti-NFTs antibodies were regionally counted using Iseki's method (Iseki et al. 1989).

Statistical Analysis

A Kruskall-Wallis analysis of variance was performed to compare: (1) LA scores, (2) (LAp-LAa)/LA scores and (3) regional scores of LA in the 30 studied areas (sum of the scores given by the two raters in each studied area) of the four groups. When a significant difference was found within the four groups, we used the nonparametric U test of Mann and Whitney to compare groups two by two.

A Spearman Rank correlation test was performed to study correlations between LA scores and (1) ages in the control group and (2) MMSE scores in the AD group.

The level of interobserver agreement for CT analysis was measured on a sample of 40 CT analyzed by four observers (DL, JPP, PV, AR) by Kappa, separately for each single area, using the Fleiss' method (Fleiss 1971; Fleiss et al. 1979). Kappa is defined as $(Po-Pe)/(1-Pe)$, where Po is the observed proportional agreement (number of all actual pairwise agreements divided by all possible pairwise agreements) and Pe is the proportion of agreements expected by chance. Kappa = 1 only when complete agreement is observed (Po = 1) and there are variations in the data (Pe < 1). Kappa cannot be defined when Pe = 1. It has been suggested in the literature (Theodossi et al. 1980) that agreement can be considered excellent when Kappa > 0.80. The level of intraobserver agreement was measured on another sample of 30 CTs analyzed again by the two observers (DL and JPP) without knowledge of their first scores, using the same Fleiss' method (Fleiss 1971; Fleiss et al. 1979).

A Kruskall-Wallis analysis of variance was performed to compare, in AD brains, the number of SP and NFT between the three groups of white matter involvement severity (Brun and Englund 1986).

Ethical Problems

None of the 98 subjects received a CT scan especially for this study. Modalities of collection, computerization and storage of data have been approved by the Regional Ethical Committee, both for patients and control subjects.

Results

Computer Tomography Scan LA Analysis

Leuko-araïosis scores were significantly different between the four groups ($p < 0.02$), with greater LA scores in AD than in PD ($p < 0.02$) and controls ($p < 0.05$) and without any significant difference between other groups (Fig. 1).

It was only possible to establish the values of the index of asymmetry in the 43 subjects (18 AD, 10 PD, 7 PSP and 8 controls) who had LA scores different from 0. The index (LAp-LAa)/LA was significantly different between the four groups ($p < 0.01$), with lower scores in PSP than in AD ($p < 0.001$), PD ($p < 0.05$) and controls ($p < 0.01$), and in PD than in AD ($p < 0.05$), without any significant difference between the other groups (Fig. 2). The regional scores of LA were significantly different between the four groups in areas "a" ($p < 0.001$), "b" ($p < 0.01$) and "h" ($p < 0.05$) (Fig. 3). In the anterior areas "a" and "b," the regional scores of LA were greater in PSP than in each of the other groups ($p < 0.001$); in the posterior area "h", the regional score of LA was greater in AD than in PD ($p < 0.01$), without any significant difference between the other groups.

Leuko-araïosis scores were correlated to age in controls ($r_s = 0.604$; $p < 0.01$), but were not correlated to MMSE scores in AD ($r_s = 0.25$; $p < 0.15$).

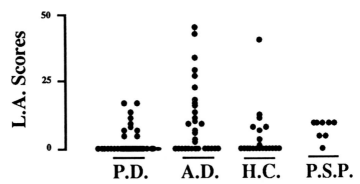

Fig. 1. Values of LA scores in subjects with Alzheimer's disease (*AD*), Parkinson's disease (*PD*), progressive supranuclear palsy (*PSP*) and healthy elderly controls (*HC*). Each point represents the "leuko-araïosis" (*LA*) score of one subject. LA scores were significantly different ($p < 0.02$) between the four groups (Kruskall-Wallis H test), with greater values in AD than in PD ($p < 0.02$) and controls ($p < 0.05$), and without any difference between the other groups (Mann and Whitney U test)

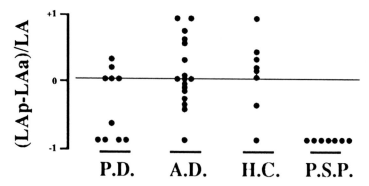

Fig. 2. The index of posterior/anterior asymmetry, (LAp-LAa)/LA, was significantly different ($p<0.01$) between the four groups (Kruskall-Wallis H test), with lower values in PSP than in AD ($p<0.001$), PD ($p<0.05$) and controls ($p<0.01$), and lower values in PD than in AD ($p<0.05$), without any significant difference between the other groups (Mann and Whitney U test)

The study of the inter- and intraobserver agreements provided the following values: for inter-observer agreement, Kappa = 0.881, and for intraobserver agreement, Kappa = 0.942 (DL) and 0.949 (JPP).

Neuropathologic Analysis

Pathologic examination of periventricular white matter was performed in two women with AD who died at ages 75 and 76; they had LA scores of 4 and 14, respectively. In both cases AD was pathologically confirmed. The degree of AD changes in these two autopsied subjects was sufficient to explain the dementia.

The white matter was characterized in both cases by diffuse myelin pallor, hyaline thickening of small vessels, and mild fibrillary astrocytosis (Fig. 4). Both patients had signs of congophilic angiopathy involving cortical vessels and sparing the white matter vessels, but neither had brain infarct or hypertensive vascular changes.

In these two patients, the number of SP did not differ regardless of the severity of the white matter changes, but the number of NFT was greater in patients with severe white matter lesions ($p<0.05$) (Fig. 5).

Fig. 3a, b. The regional scores of LA in 15 areas in each hemisphere of 4 CT slices were significantly different between the 4 groups (Kruskall-Wallis H test) in areas "a" ($p<0.001$), "b" ($p<0.01$) and "h" ($p<0.05$). In areas "a" and "b," values were greater in PSP than in all other groups ($p<0.001$); in area "h," the regional score of LA was significantly greater in AD than in PD ($p<0.01$), without any significant difference between the other groups (Mann and Whitney U test)

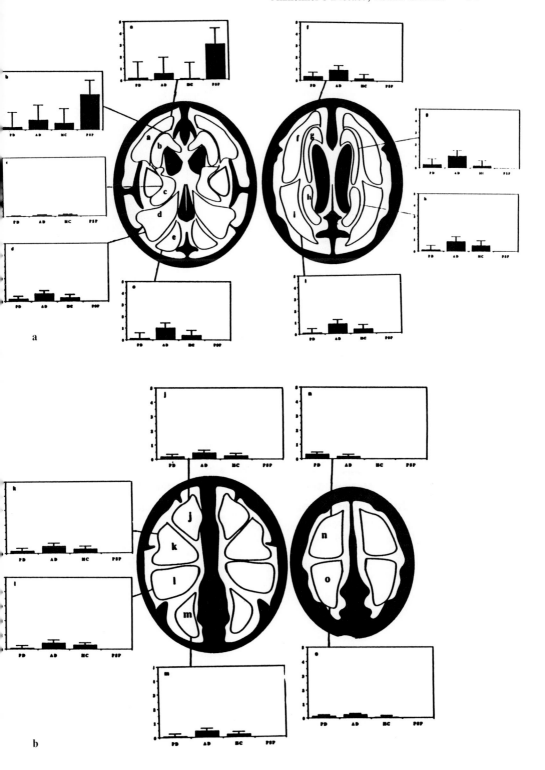

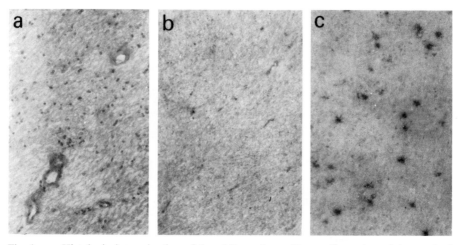

Fig. 4a–c. Histological examination of the white matter. **a** Hemoxylin-eosin staining method: hyaline mural thickening of small cerebral arteries. **b** Spielmeyer staining method: diffuse myelin pallor. **c** Anti-GFAP immunohistochemistry: mild fibrillary astrocytosis

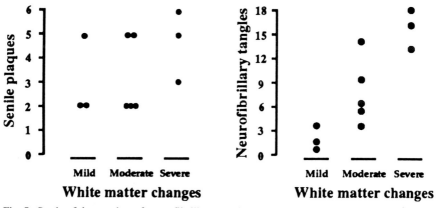

Fig. 5. Study of the number of neurofibrillary tangles (NFT) and of the number of senile plaques (SP) (using Iseki's criteria (1989)) as a function of the severity of white matter lesions [using Brun and Englund's criteria (1986)]. The number of SP was not different regardless of the severity of the white matter changes, but the number of NFT was greater in patients with severe white matter lesions ($p < 0.05$)

Discussion

Our study revealed that: (1) in AD, LA scores were greater than in control subjects, (2) in AD, LA was more prominent in posterior periventricular areas, whereas in PD and PSP, LA was more prominent in anterior periventricular areas; (3) in two patients with AD and LA, autopsy revealed diffuse white matter pallor, limited hyaline thickening of small white matter vessels, and mild fibrillary astrocytosis, without any infarction or hypertensive change; and (4) changes were more severe in white matter close to cortical areas with a great density of NFT but not to cortical areas with a great density of SP.

Previous studies, except that by Rezek et al. (1987), did not attempt to quantify the severity of LA; most authors separated subjects with LA from subjects without LA. To our knowledge this type of study of LA in PD and PSP has never been performed, and no previous studies have attempted to account for the topography of LA.

In AD we found greater LA scores than in control subjects. Confirming previous studies (Rezek et al. 1987; Akaron-Peretz et al. 1988), ours also suggested that factors other than hypertension, diabetes mellitus or cardiac diseases could be associated with LA, and that neuropathological lesions of AD might be one of them. The greater LA scores in AD when compared to PD, without any difference between PD, PSP and controls, suggested that this factor of LA is more severe or more widespread in AD than in PD, PSP and normal aging. Nevertheless this factor is not specific to AD, since LA was found in PD, PSP and controls.

In PD we found a slight predominance of LA in anterior areas, which are sometimes clinically affected in PD (Taylor et al. 1986), though available data are quite discordant. In PSP we found a strong predominance of LA in anterior areas, which usually are severely affected, as suggested by clinical (Cambier et al. 1985) and metabolic studies (D'Antona et al. 1985; Goffinet et al. 1989). Thus, our radiological study suggested that, if an intrinsic factor of LA was present in the four groups, it was more severe and more posterior in AD. None of the four neuropathologic lesions of AD (neuronal loss, NFT, SP and amyloid angiopathy) is specific (Delacourte et al. 1988); the greater severity of these lesions in AD when compared to PD, PSP and normal aging might explain why LA is more severe in AD.

If NFT and SP have the same location in the AD group and other groups (Delacourte et al. 1988), they cannot be direct factors of LA, since we found differences in LA locations between the four groups. Our two autopsied patients had signs of amyloid angiopathy only in cortical vessels but not in the white matter, as was previously reported in five cases by Rezek et al. (1987). This suggests that amyloid angiopathy might not be a direct factor of LA. Moreover, the frequency of LA in AD is usually high (Rezek et al. 1987), though neuropathological data usually reveal no sign of amyloid angiopathy in the white matter in either AD (Brun and Englund 1986; Englund et al. 1988, Bergeron et al. 1987) or in primary amyloid angiopathies (Bogucki et al. 1988; Masuda et al. 1988). However, since amyloid angiopathy increases with age (Masuda et al. 1988) and is usually prominent in posterior cortical and leptomeningeal vessels (Masuda et al. 1988), gray matter neuronal loss due to the cortical lesions of amyloid angiopathy cannot be excluded. Moreover, the cortical blood supply and the subjacent U fibers are richly served by collaterals, so that if a cortical vessel with amyloid is occluded the adjacent gray matter and U fibers may be spread by adequate collateral flow. The white matter served by the same artery may suffer ischemic damage since once the artery penetrates the white matter it has no collaterals (Hachinski et al. 1987). Nevertheless, the mechanism of "incomplete infarction" previously suggested by Brun and Englund (1986; Englund et al.

1988) cannot explain why LA is more prominent in anterior areas in PD and PSP, because cortical amyloid angiopathy has the same location in AD and normal aging and usually only differs in its severity. Thus, the differences in the location of LA that we observed between the other four groups cannot support the mechanism suggested by Brun and Englund (1986; Englund et al. 1988) to explain a white matter disorder in AD. Differences in the location of LA between the four groups might more probably be explained by a decrease of myelin density secondary to the Wallerian degeneration due to the gray matter disorder (Ball 1989), which is more widespread in AD than in PD, PSP and normal aging, and probably more anterior in PSP (Cambier et al. 1985; D'Antona et al. 1985; Goffinet et al. 1989) and perhaps in PD (Taylor et al. 1986).

Our study suggested a relationship between neuronal loss – subcortical in PD and PSP and cortical in AD – and white matter lesions. If LA is secondary to a neuronal drop-out, we would expect the eight control patients with LA to have cognitive impairment; however, their neuropsychological examinations were limited to the MMSE (Folstein et al. 1975), which might have an inadequate sensitivity to detect "preclinical" AD. Moreover, we found a trend toward a negative correlation between LA scores and MMSE in AD, but it did not reach a statistical level of significancy. This point is of major interest since De La Monte (1989) suggested, from neuropathological data, that white matter lesions in "preclinical" AD might precede cortical lesions. Do these changes herald the subsequent development of dementia? Only further longitudinal studies can answer this question.

Acknowledgements. We thank C. Caullet, MD; A. Fauquette, MD; Y. Gaudet, MD; and G. Gozet, MD, for their help.

References

Adams RD, Victor M (1985) Principles of neurology, 3rd edn. McGraw-Hill, New York, pp 874–879

Aharon-Peretz J, Cummings JL, Hill MA (1988) Vascular dementia and dementia of the Alzheimer type. Cognition, ventricular size and leuco-araïosis. Arch Neurol 45:719–721

Ball MJ (1989) "Leukoaraiosis" explained. Lancet i:612–613

Bergeron C, Ranalli PJ, Miceli PN (1987) Amyloid angiopathy in Alzheimer's disease. Can J Neurol Sci 14:564–569

Blin J, Baron JC, Dubois B, et al. (1989) Depression of regional brain energy metabolism in progressive supranuclear palsy and clinico-metabolic correlations. J Cereb Blood Flow Metab 9:S21

Bogucki A, Papierz W, Szymanska R, Staniaszczyk R (1988) Cerebral amyloid angiopathy with attenuation of the white matter on CT scans: subcortical arteriosclerotic encephalopathy (Binswanger) in a normotensive patient. J Neurol 235:435–437

Brun A, Englund E (1986) A white matter disorder in dementia of the Alzheimer type: a pathoanatomical study. Ann Neurol 19:253–262

Cambier J, Masson M, Viader F, et al. (1985) Le syndrome frontal de la paralysie supranucléaire progressive. Rev Neurol (Paris) 141:528–536

D'Antona R, Baron JC, Samson Y, et al. (1985) Subcortical dementia: frontal cortex hypometabolism detected by positron tomography in patients with progressive supranuclear palsy. Brain 108:785–799

Delacourte A, Lenders MB, Défossez A, et al. (1988) Neuropathologie et neurobiologie de la maladie d'Alzheimer. In: Leys D, Petit H (eds) La maladie d'Alzheimer et ses limites. Masson, Paris, pp 103–113

De la Monte SM (1989) Quantification of cerebral atrophy in preclinical and end-stage Alzheimer's disease. Ann Neurol 25:450–459

De Reuck J, Crevits L, De Coster W, et al. (1980) Pathogenesis of Binswanger's chronic subcortical encephalopathy. Neurology 30:920–928

Englund E, Brun A, Alling C (1988) White matter changes in dementia of Alzheimer's type: biochemical and neuropathological correlates. Brain 111:1425–1439

Fleiss JL (1971) Measuring nominal scale agreement among many raters. Psychol Bull 76:378–382

Fleiss JL, Nee JCM, Landis JR (1979) Large sample variance of Kappa in the case of different sets of raters. Psychol Bull 86:974–977

Folstein MF, Folstein SE, Mc Hugh PR (1975) "Mini-Mental state." A practical method for grading the cognitive state of patients for the clinician. J Psychiat Res 12:189–198

Goffinet AM, De Volder AG, Gillain C, et al. (1989) Positron tomography demonstrates frontal lobe hypometabolism in progressive supranuclear palsy. Ann Neurol 25:131–139

Gupta SR, Naheedy MH, Young JC, et al. (1988) Periventricular white matter changes and dementia. Clinical, neuropsychological, radiological and pathological correlations. Arch Neurol 45:637–641

Hachinski VC, Potter P, Merskey H (1987) Leuko-araïosis. Arch Neurol 44:21–23

Huang K, Wu L, Luo Y (1985) Binswanger's disease: progressive subcortical encephalopathy or multi-infarct dementia? Can J Neurol Sci 12:88–94

Inzitari D, Diaz F, Fox A, et al. (1987) Vascular risk factors and leuco-araïosis. Arch Neurol 44:42–47

Iseki E, Matsushita M, Kosaka K, et al. (1989) Distribution and morphology of brain stem plaques in Alzheimer's disease. Acta Neuropathol 78:131–136

Kinkel WR, Jacobs L, Polachini I, et al. (1985) Subcortical arteriosclerotic encephalopathy (Binswanger's disease): computed tomographic, nuclear magnetic resonance, clinical correlations. Arch Neurol 42:951–959

Leys D, Pruvo J-P, Petit H, et al. (1989a) Maladie d'Alzheimer: analyse statistique des résultats du scanner X. Rev Neurol (Paris) 145:134–139

Leys D, Steinling M, Petit H, et al. (1989b) Maladie d'Alzheimer: Etude par tomographie d'émission monophotonique (Hm Pao Tc 99m). Rev Neurol (Paris) 145:443–450

Loeb C, Gandolfo C (1983) Diagnostic evaluation of degenerative and vascular dementia. Stroke 14:399–401

Loizou LA, Kendall BE, Marshall J (1981) Subcortical arteriosclerotic encephalopathy: a clinical and radiological investigation. J Neurol Neurosurg Psychiatry 44:294–304

Masuda J, Tanaka K, Ueda K, Omae T (1988) Autopsy study of incidence and distribution of cerebral amyloid angiopathy in Hisayama, Japan. Stroke 19:205–210

Mc Kahnn G, Drachman D, Folstein M, et al. (1984) Clinical diagnosis of Alzheimer's disease: Report of the NINCDS ADRDA work group under the auspices of Departement of Health and Human Services task force on Alzheimer's disease. Neurology 34:939–944

Rezek DL, Morris JC, Fulling KH, et al. (1987) Periventricular white matter lucencies in senile dementia of the Alzheimer type and in normal aging. Neurology 37:1365–1368

Steingart A, Hachinski VC, Lau C, et al. (1987a) Cognitive and neurologic findings in subjects with diffuse white matter lucencies on computed tomographic scan (leuko-araïosis). Arch Neurol 44:32–35

Steingart A, Hachinski VC, Lau C, et al. (1987b) Cognitive and neurologic findings in demented patients with diffuse white matter lucencies on computed tomographic scan (leuko-araïosis). Arch Neurol 44:36–39

Taylor AE, Saint-Cyr JA, Lang AE (1986) Frontal lobe dysfunction in Parkinson's disease. The cortical focus of neostriatal outflow. Brain 109:845–883

Theodossi A, Skene AM, Portmann B, et al. (1980) Observer variation assessment in liver biopsies including analysis by Kappa statistics. Gastroenterology 79:232–241

Topographical Comparison of Lesions in Trisomy 21 and Alzheimer's Disease: A Study with PET, Anatomical and Neuropathological Investigations

M. B. Schapiro, J. V. Haxby, C. L. Grady, and S. I. Rapoport

Summary

Recent evidence suggests that Alzheimer's disease (AD) is a clinically heterogeneous disorder and that specific subgroups exist. A human model of AD exists that avoids such problems as heterogeneity. Down's syndrome (DS), trisomy 21, is a genetic disorder in which an extra portion of chromosome 21 leads to mental retardation, short stature, and phenotypic abnormalities. DS subjects over 35 years of age demonstrate neuropathological and neurochemical defects postmortem which are virtually indistinguishable from those found in brain of AD patients, as well as a universal cognitive deterioration and a 20%–30% prevalence of dementia. In older DS subjects and AD patients, positron emission tomography (PET) shows identical patterns of abnormal glucose metabolism, selectively involving association areas of frontal, parietal and temporal neocortices, but sparing primary sensory and motor regions. In demented DS as well as AD patients, furthermore, quantitative computer assisted tomography (CT) indicates accelerated neuronal loss and brain atrophy.

As a potential use of the DS model, we have observed a case of DS with dementia but without mental retardation. This case suggests that expression of dementia in DS can involve genes on chromosome 21 other than in the "obligatory" distal segment of the q arm. Alternatively, differential expression of genes on the q arm of chromosome 21 might cause dementia without the phenotypic features and mental retardation.

Introduction

A problem in genetic studies of Alzheimer's disease (AD) is the possible etiologic heterogeneity of the disorder, including the uncertainty as to whether there are multiple genetic or nongenetic causes. Recent evidence suggests that AD is a clinically heterogeneous disorder and that specific subtypes exist (Kaye et al. 1988). A human model of AD exists that avoids this problem of heterogeneity. Down syndrome (DS), trisomy 21, is a genetic disorder in which an extra portion of chromosome 21 leads to mental retardation, short stature, and other phenotypic abnormalities (Rahmani et al. 1989). Further, DS subjects over age 35 years demonstrate neuropathological (Mann et al. 1984; Ball et al. 1986) and neuro-chemical (Yates et al. 1983) defects postmortem which are virtually indistinguish-able from those found in brains of AD patients, as well as a universal cognitive deterioration and a 20% – 30% prevalence of dementia (Schapiro et al. 1989 b). Other evidence also links the two disorders: the incidence of DS is higher in families of AD patients than in the general population (Heston et al. 1981; Hey-man et al. 1983); a restriction fragment polymorphism from chromosome 21 segregates with early-onset familial AD (St. George-Hyslop et al. 1987); the gene coding for the precursor protein of beta-amyloid has been assigned to chromo-some 21 (Goldgaber et al. 1987; Tanzi et al. 1987); and the expression of the amyloid precursor protein mRNA lacking the protease inhibitor domain is de-pressed in both aged DS and AD brains in neocortical association regions (Neve et al. 1988).

Although prior reports had considered the relation of DS and AD, many methodological issues were ignored. DS subjects were included with significant medical illnesses, such as hypothyroidism and congenital heart disease. Medica-tions, such as psychotropics, were not discontinued during testing. Many subjects were recruited from institutions, where educational and training opportunities were limited. Karyotypes were not described. The level of mental retardation was not characterized, and, most importantly, the presence or absence of dementia was often not described.

Because of opportunities available with newer techniques, including positron emission tomography (PET) with [^{18}F]fluoro-2-deoxy-D-glucose (18FDG) to study brain metabolism, and quantitative computed assisted tomography (CT) to study brain anatomy, our laboratory formulated a program in 1983 to address age changes and mental retardation in DS adults, in concert with our study of AD. Specific questions were addressed. What are the cognitive deficits in adults with DS and how does one distinguish dementia from mental retardation? Is there brain atrophy in young or older DS adults? Are there changes in brain metabolism in young or older adults with DS? Do different parts of chromosome 21 determine dementia as opposed to mental retardation in DS? What hypotheses does DS allow one to generate about the pathogenesis and course of AD?

Methods

To avoid previously mentioned methodological problems, we studied only care-fully screened, healthy, noninstitutionalized DS subjects, whose mental status and cognitive deficits could be quantified (Schapiro et al. 1987 b). All subjects (except one to be discussed separately) were trisomy 21 karyotype. In order to distinguish mental retardation from dementia, the DS subjects were divided into those 18 – 40 years (mentally retarded but presumably free of Alzheimer's neuropathology) and those over 40 years (with Alzheimer's neuropathology and possible demen-tia).

Neuropsychological assessment was performed using standardized tests. The Peabody Picture Vocabulary Test-Revised (Dunn and Dunn 1981) and Stanford-

Binet Intelligence Scale (Terman and Merrill 1973) were used to assess general intelligence. Visuospatial ability was evaluated with the Block Pattern Subtest of the Hiskey Nebraska Test of Learning Aptitude (Hiskey 1955), the WISC-R Block Design Subtest (Wechsler 1974), and the Extended Block Design Test (Haxby 1989). Attention was assessed using forward digit span, object pointing span, and block tapping span (Haxby 1989). Visual recognition memory was measured with a design span (Haxby 1989).

Noncontrast CT scans of brain were performed with a GE 8800 CT scanner (General Electric Co., Milwaukee, WI), for which full width half maximum equaled 1 mm. Serial slices, each 10 mm thick and separated from adjacent slices by 7 mm (center to center), were taken parallel to and from 0 to 110 mm above the inferior orbitomeatal (IOM) line. Analysis was limited to levels 30–80 mm above the IOM line. A semi-automated method of analysis was used. CT data were stored on magnetic tape in digital form, and were analyzed on a PDP 11/34 computer (Digital Equipment Corporation, Maynard, MA) with a DeAnza Picture Display Monitor (Gould Inc., Freemont, CA). An image-processing program (CATSEG) allowed determination of the number of pixels of gray matter, white matter, and cerebrospinal fluid (CSF). In addition, regions of interest (ROIs) were outlined around the ventricles, using a digitalizing graphics tablet and a light pen. Intracranial surface area was derived with an automatic edge-finding procedure (Schwartz et al. 1985).

The regional cerebral metabolic rates for glucose (rCMRglc) were measured in the resting state using 18FDG and a PET tomograph. Subjects received 5 mCi 18FDG intravenously and then spent 45 min in a darkened and quiet room with eyes patched and ears occluded. Initial studies were performed with an ECAT II PET tomograph (ORTEC, Life Sciencs, Oak Ridge, TN), which used a calculated attenuation correction program. Seven serial slices were collected (Schapiro et al., 1987 b). Later studies were performed with a multislice PET scanner (Scanditronix PC-1024-7B, Sweden), using a measured attenuation correction (Schapiro et al. 1989 a). After comparing PET images with anatomic sections from an atlas of a human brain, a "height above the IOM line" of the slice in the atlas was assigned to each PET slice. Anatomic regions of interest in the pET slices were then identified.

Neuropsychology

Some authors believe that it is difficult to diagnose dementia in mentally retarded subjects. However, we believe that the distinction can be made using specific diagnostic criteria. In our laboratory, the diagnosis of dementia in DS was made using modified criteria from the Diagnostic and Statistical Manual, which specified an acquired, progressive loss of intellectual function, such as loss of daily living and vocational skills, memory impairment, reduced speech and comprehension, and personality change (Schapiro et al. 1987 b). The diagnosis was based on narrative reports of caregivers or employers, which were supplemented by clinical examination and bedside mental status tests. Previous medical and psychological reports were reviewed when available. Interrater reliability for the diagnosis of dementia was assessed in our subjects with a Kappa statistic (Bartko and Carpenter 1976). For two physicians independently rating each subject, the Kappa was 0.828 ($p < 0.001$), suggesting that agreement was better than by chance (Schapiro et al. 1989b). Autopsy of each of three older demented subjects (55-year-old woman; 47- and 66-year-old men) showed extensive neuropathological changes of AD.

Though all DS adults develop the neuropathological changes of AD, only a minority of older DS adults demonstrate clinically significant dementia (Wisniewski et al. 1985). This discrepancy may be due to the insensitivity of caregiver reports and clinical examination to the early behavioral changes (dementia) associated with Alzheimer's neuropathology, suggesting that formal neuropsychological testing reveals earlier changes (Haxby 1989).

Therefore, we designed a battery of neuropsychological tests to examine patterns of age-related neuropsychological changes in older DS adults with and without dementia. Overall ability, using the Peabody Picture Vocabulary Test, was 6.8 ± 3.1 (mean $\pm$ SD) years in 19 young DS subjects, 4.7 ± 1.5 years in six nondemented old DS subjects, and 2.3 ± 0.4 years in four demented old DS subjects (Haxby 1989). Mean mental ages on the Stanford Binet Test were similar. The demented older DS group differed significantly ($p < 0.05$) from the young DS group on both measures. However, the nondemented older DS group did not differ from the younger subjects, "suggesting that the nondemented older subjects probably had mental abilities as young adults that were equivalent to the young DS subjects current abilities" (Haxby 1989).

Other cognitive tasks were specifically evaluated, including immediate memory, long-term memory, language, and visuospatial ability. Relative to the young DS subjects, the six nondemented older DS subjects demonstrated a distinctive pattern of spared abilities (such as immediate memory span and language) and diminished abilities (such as long-term memory and visuospatial construction). On the other hand, of the four demented older DS subjects, two scored lower than the young DS group on all functions. The other two subjects also scored at the lower end or below on immediate memory, long-term memory, and visuospatial construction, though language scores were within the young DS group range.

Thus, these findings suggest that cognitive changes occur with age in DS, but are more severe in demented as compared to nondemented older subjects. A distinctive pattern of age-related deficits occurs in nondemented older DS subjects, which resembles the pattern seen in early to intermediate dementia of the Alzheimer type in premorbidly normal subjects. The pattern of cognitive failure in the demented older subjects is more global. In addition, dementia, based on caregiver reports and clinical examination, occurs only in a fraction of older DS adults.

Quantitative Computer Assisted Tomography

Previous pathological studies have suggested that brain weight in young DS adults is less than normal, but extreme microcephaly is rare (Solitare and Lamarche 1967). From such pathological studies it is unclear whether cerebral atrophy occurs in young DS subjects (Burger and Vogel 1973; Wisniewski et al. 1985). Since CT measures of brain avoid postmortem problems (Schwartz et al. 1985), we used CT to evaluate the dimensions of brain, CSF and cerebral ventricles in DS subjects.

Mean total intracranial volume was significantly less in 18 young DS adults than in 16 young healthy controls, 1067 cm^3 versus 1241 cm^3 ($p < 0.05$). When normalized to height (to correct for the shorter stature in DS), the difference was no longer shown. In addition, there was no significant difference in CSF or ventricular volume, either directly or after normalization to seven-slice intracranial volume (Schapiro et al. 1987a).

Although AD is accompanied by progressive cerebral atrophy on CT (Luxenberg et al. 1987), it is not known to what extent demented older DS adults have cortical atrophy. Therefore, we used quantitative CT, in cross-sectional and longitudinal analyses, to examine whether differences in brain morphology help to distinguish dementia from mental retardation.

In cross-sectional studies, comparison between 5 nondemented older and 12 young adult DS subjects showed no significant difference in volume of CSF; 18.6 ± 14.0 cm^3 versus 25.5 ± 13.4 cm^3 (mean $\pm$ SD, $p > 0.05$) (Schapiro et al. 1989b). However, significant increases in CSF volume were shown between 3 demented older and 12 young DS subjects (50.9 ± 11.2 versus 25.5 ± 13.4 cm^3), and between 3 demented and 5 nondemented older subjects (50.9 ± 11.2 versus 18.6 ± 14.0 cm^3). In addition, total ventricular volume was increased by 85% and 102% in the demented as compared to the young and nondemented older groups, respectively (although these differences failed to reach significance).

In longitudinal studies, CT scans were separated by an average of 43 months in the 12 young DS subjects, 20 months in the 5 nondemented old DS subjects, and 22 months in the 3 demented older DS subjects. A slight increase for rate of change of CSF volume was observed between the young and nondemented old DS groups, -1.32 ± 1.90 versus 2.50 ± 1.81 cm^3/year. Greater rates of change of CSF volume were noted between the young and demented older DS groups, -1.32 ± 1.90 versus 10.90 ± 4.32 cm^3/year ($p < 0.05$). These rates of change for CSF volume in the demented old DS group also differed significantly from those in the nondemented old DS group.

Thus, in DS, smaller brains reflect a smaller stature and a smaller cranial vault present in this syndrome. This is similar to findings in male and female controls, where it is established that brain weight is proportional to body height (Dekaban and Sadowsky 1978). No cerebral atrophy occurs in young DS adults, suggesting that the mental retardation is related to inherent cerebral dysfunction and not to acquired cerebral atrophy. Further, cross-sectional and longitudinal studies differentiate nondemented and demented older DS subjects. Demented older DS adults have accelerated brain atrophy, indicating that neuronal loss is critical for dementia.

Positron Emission Tomography

As a reflection of neuronal activity, cerebral metabolism and blood flow have been studied in young adults with DS (Fazekas et al. 1958; Lassen et al. 1966; Risberg 1980; Schwartz et al. 1983; Melamed et al. 1987). We reevaluated brain metabolism using PET and 18FDG to learn if there are differences in absolute cerebral metabolic rates between young DS adults and age-matched controls, and if there are changes in pattern of metabolism prior to the development of Alzheimer's neuropathology in old DS subjects.

There was no significant difference in global or gray matter rCMRglc between young DS and control subjects. Global CMRglc was 8.76 ± 0.76 (mean $\pm$ SD) in 14 young DS adults versus 8.74 ± 1.19 mg/100 g per minute in 13 young controls. There was preservation of rCMRglc in both neocortical association areas and primary motor and sensory areas. Reference ratios (rCMRglc/global CMRglc) also did not differ between groups. In addition, within the DS group, subjects with mental ages over 8 years did not differ from those with mental ages less than 8 years for any rCMRglc ratio (Schapiro et al. 1989 a).

Thus, young DS adults (< 40 years and without dementia) do not have altered cerebral glucose metabolism, at rest and with reduced sensory input. In addition, reference ratios show no consistent difference in the intrahemispheric distribution of rCMRglc compared to controls. The lack of selective metabolic involvement of neocortex in young DS adults differs from the pattern seen in demented older DS adults (see below). Finally, metabolic differences cannot identify young DS adults "at risk" for later Alzheimer's neuropathology.

Brain metabolism and blood flow have also been studied in older DS adults. Though not specifically looked for, age-related differences in blood flow and metabolism were not shown, and dementia was not examined. In our laboratory, PET with 18FDG was used to determine if there are age-related differences in brain glucose metabolism in DS and to determine if differences in brain metabolism help to distinguish dementia from mental retardation in DS adults over 35 years.

Table 1 shows representative absolute values of rCMRglc for young, nondemented old, and demented old DS groups. For both association and primary neocortex, nondemented old DS subjects had glucose metabolic values that were more similar to those of the young DS subjects, as indicated by the lack of significant differences between the nondemented old and young DS subjects. On the other hand, demented older DS subjects had significantly lower values of rCMRglc than young DS subjects, with the greatest reductions in association neocortex. The demented older group also had significantly lower values of rCMRglc in association neocortex in comparison to nondemented older DS subjects. Thus, decreased brain metabolism is seen only in older DS subjects with dementia.

The intrahemispheric pattern of glucose metabolism was examined with the ratio of parietal association cortex to sensorimotor primary cortex. There was no significant difference between 15 young and 4 nondemented older DS subjects (0.94 ± 0.01 versus 0.92 ± 0.03) (mean $\pm$ SEM). However, the ratio in 3 demented older DS subjects (0.80 ± 0.01) was significantly less (without overlap) than in

Table 1. Regional cerebral metabolic rate for glucose (rCMRglc) in young, nondemented old, and demented old DS subjects. Values are mean ± standard error. Differences between mean values in DS groups were compared with a one-way ANOVA. Post hoc comparisons were performed with Bonferroni t tests ($p < 0.05$)

	Young DS (15)	Nondemented old DS (4)	Demented old DS (3)
Association neocortex			
Parietal	7.14 ± 0.24 [a]	6.29 ± 0.51	4.19 ± 0.49 [b, c]
Lateral temporal	5.65 ± 0.18	5.07 ± 0.27	3.68 ± 0.33 [b, c]
Primary neocortex			
Sensorimotor	7.58 ± 0.25	6.87 ± 0.59	5.21 ± 0.56 [b]
Occipital	6.43 ± 0.21	6.30 ± 0.15	4.92 ± 0.64 [b]

[a] Mean + SEM (mg/100 g per minute)
[b] Differs from mean in young DS group ($p < 0.05$)
[c] Differs from mean in nondemented old DS group ($p < 0.05$)

both the young and nondemented older DS groups. Similar changes were shown for the ratio of temporal association cortex to primary occipital cortex.

Thus, glucose metabolism is preserved in older DS subjects without clinical dementia. Glucose metabolism is reduced in older DS subjects with clinical dementia. The metabolism is not uniformly reduced, however, with specific involvement of parietal-temporal association neocortices. This relatively greater involvement of parietal-temporal regions is specific for older DS subjects with dementia.

Hypothesis

Previously, it was thought paradoxical that only 20%–30% of older DS subjects were demented despite the universal presence of neuropathological changes of AD after age 35 years. Explanations for the discrepancy included the difficulty of diagnosing dementia in mentally retarded subjects, the delay of age-of-onset of dementia, the variable clinical course of dementia, and the resistance to the development of dementia in a less sensitive brain. We also note that only a fraction of our older DS subjects are demented, despite the likelihood, given their poor performance on standardized neuropsychological tests, that all have neuropathological changes of AD.

Though some authors believe that the density of senile plaques and neurofibrillary tangles correlates with the severity of dementia (Wisniewski et al. 1985), others disagree (Ropper and Williams 1980). However, one study showed that even in brains with more than 20 senile plaques or neurofibrillary tangles per high power field, only 13 of 28 subjects had a history of dementia (Wisniewski et al. 1985).

This suggests that an additional factor contributes to the expression of dementia in older DS subjects who show measureable cognitive decline. This factor may be the additional appearance of large numbers of neurofibrillary tangles and cell loss, which together may occur 10–20 years later than the appearance of large numbers of senile plaques (Haberland 1969; Burger and Vogel 1973; Mann and Esiri 1989).

We hypothesize that a cognitive decline in older DS subjects occurs in two stages which can be separated by as much as 20 years. First, there is a reduction in cognitive performance on standardized neuropsychological tests, perhaps reflective of poorer processing skills. The reduction correlates with significant accumulations of senile plaques, but neurofibrillary tangle accumulation, cell loss and cerebral atrophy have not yet occurred. This interpretation is supported by the absence of a change in ventricular volume on quantitative CT and normal brain metabolism on PET scanning in our nondemented older DS group, as compared to the young DS group.

In the second stage, there is additional loss of overlearned behaviors, leading to deterioration in social, occupational and adaptive skills and a characteristic dementia. Concurrently, accumulations of neurofibrillary tangles and accelerated cell loss are occurring. Cell death is evidenced by progressive brain atrophy on quantitative CT and decreased brain metabolism, as seen in our demented older DS group.

Thus, our results suggest that progressive brain atrophy and reduced brain metabolism occur only in demented old DS subjects, and that quantitative CT and PET with 18FDG can help to distinguish dementia from lesser cognitive decline in older DS subjects.

Mosaic/Translocation Down's Syndrome

When dementia was described previously in DS, such cases were mentally retarded. Thus, the relation of mental retardation and dementia has not been defined. We had the opportunity to study a patient of DS who developed dementia without mental retardation.

The subject was a 45-year-old woman who presented with a 2-year history of dementia. As an infant, her physician suggested that she might have DS, but this was not followed up. She graduated from public high school with average grades and was employed for the next 25 years as a teller and clerk-typist until onset of her dementia. Cognitive decline continued over the next 2.5 years. Examination showed normal stature and head circumference. Stigmata of DS included brachycephaly, midfacial hypoplasia, bilateral clinodactyly, and an R Simian crease. There were no Brushfield spots, small ears, enlarged tongue, or heart murmur.

Peripheral blood chromosome analysis showed a single cell (1/100) with a missing number 21 and an atypical small metacentric with banding consistent with a t(21;21) rearrangement. The other cells with 46 chromosomes appeared to have two normal 21 chromosomes and no abnormalities of the other autosomes or sex chromosomes. Two Giemsa-trypsin banded karyotypes were unremarkable. A repeat high resolution study of peripheral blood was normal. Following skin punch biopsy, one of two fibroblast cultures showed a 46,XX,−21, + t(21;21) translocation trisomy 21 karyotype in all cells. In the other fibroblast culture, all cells had two normal appearing number 21 chromosomes, and a normal chromosome count of 46. Examination of both parents showed normal peripheral blood karyotypes.

Initial neuropsychologic assessment showed a WAIS Verbal IQ score (Wechsler 1955) of 85, which is within the normal range. On the other hand, her initial score on the Mattis Dementia Scale (Mattis 1976) was 121 (normal >136), indicative of mild dementia. Subsequent neuropsychologic assessment showed decline in cognitive abilities. Furthermore she had dilated ventricles on quantitative CT and reduced parietal and temporal glucose metabolism on PET scanning with 18FDG as seen in AD patients.

Thus, AD in DS may occur without mental retardation. In light of the normal body growth, absence of mental retardation, and minimal physical stigmata of DS in our case, it is suggested that the typical phenotypic expression of DS is not necessary for the late expression of dementia in DS. Development of dementia in DS may involve genes in regions of chromosome 21 other than the obligatory DS region (Rahmani et al. 1989), since genes in this region did not appear to be expressed in this case. Our chromosomal findings in this case suggest that this region is not on the short arm of chromosome 21 and that it could be proximal to the q 22.1 band. This is supportive of the studies by St. George-Hyslop et al. (1987) suggesting that there is a locus for susceptibility to familial Alzheimer's disease on the proximal portion of the q arm of chromosome 21.

Conclusions

In DS an extra portion of chromosome 21 results in a dementia syndrome that is phenotypically identical to AD in premorbidly normal individuals. This dementia can be reliably diagnosed in DS despite the mental retardation. However, more sensitive formal neuropsychological tests are needed to detect lesser cognitive decline in nondemented older DS subjects. Identical patterns of abnormal glucose metabolism, selectively involving association areas of parietal and temporal neocortices, are present in older DS subjects with dementia and premorbidly normal AD patients. Further, progressive brain atrophy is present in demented DS as well as premorbidly normal AD patients. Both quantitative CT and PET scanning with 18FDG can distinguish dementia from lesser cognitive decline in older DS. Finally, dementia in DS can occur without mental retardation, suggesting that expression of dementia may involve genes on chromosome 21 other than in the obligatory distal segment of the q arm. Further research may show the importance of chromosome 21 for the study of AD and how abnormal excess or differential expression of different genes on this chromosome leads to different features, such as mental retardation or dementia.

References

Ball MJ, Schapiro MB, Rapoport SI (1986) Neuropathological relationships between Down's syndrome and senile dementia Alzheimer type. In: Epstein CJ (ed) The neurobiology of Down syndrome. New York, Raven Press, pp 45–58

Bartko JJ, Carpenter WT (1976) On the methods and theory of reliability. J Nerv Ment Dis 163:307–317

Burger PC, Vogel FS (1973) The development of the pathologic changes of Alzheimer's disease and senile dementia in patients with Down's syndrome. Am J Pathol 73:457–476

Dekaban AS, Sadowsky D (1978) Changes in brain weights during the span of human life: relation of brain weights to body heights and body weights. Ann Neurol 4:345–356

Dunn LM, Dunn LM (1981) Peabody Picture Vocabulary Test-Revised. American Guidance Service, Circle Pines, New Mexico

Fazekas JF, Ehrmantraut WR, Shea JG, Kleh J (1958) Cerebral hemodynamics and metabolism in mental deficiency. Neurology 8:558–560

Goldgaber D, Lerman MI, McBride OW, Saffiotti U, Gajdusek DC (1987) Characterization and chromosomal localization of a cDNA encoding brain amyloid of Alzheimer's disease. Science 235:877–879

Haberland C (1969) Alzheimer's disease in Down syndrome: clinical-neuropathological observations. Acta Neurol Belg 69:369–380

Haxby JV (1989) Neuropsychological evaluation of adults with Down's syndrome: patterns of selective impairment in non-demented old adults. J Ment Defic Res 33:193–210

Heston LL, Mastri AR, Anderson VE, White J (1981) Dementia of the Alzheimer type: clinical genetics, natural history, and associated conditions. Arch Gen Psychiat 38:1085–1090

Heyman A, Wilkinson WE, Hurwitz BJ, Schmechel D, Sigmon AH, Weinberg T, Helms MJ, Swift M (1983) Alzheimer's disease: genetic aspects and associated clinical disorders. Ann Neurol 14:507–515

Hiskey MS (1955) Hiskey-Nebraska Test of Learning Aptitude. College View Printers, Lincoln, Nebraska

Kaye JA, May C, Daly E, Atack JR, Sweeney DJ, Luxenberg JS, Kay AD, Kaufman S, Milstein S, Friedland RP, Rapoport SI (1988) Cerebrospinal fluid monoamine markers are decreased in dementia of the Alzheimer's type with extrapyramidal features. Neurology 38:554–557

Lassen NA, Christensen S, Hoedt-Rasmussen K, Stewart BM (1966) Cerebral oxygen consumption in Down's syndrome. Arch Neurol 15:595–602

Luxenberg JS, Haxby JV, Creasey H, Sundaram M, Rapoport SI (1987) Rate of ventricular enlargement in dementia of the Alzheimer type correlates with rate of neuropsychological deterioration. Neurology 37:1135–1140

Mann DMA, Esiri MM (1989) The pattern of acquisition of plaques and tangles in the brains of patients under 50 years of age with Down's syndrome. J Neurol Sci 89:169–179

Mann DMA, Yates PO, Marcyniuk B (1984) Alzheimer's presenile dementia, senile dementia of Alzheimer type and Down's syndrome in middle age from an age-related continuum of pathological changes. Neuropathol Appl Neurobiol 10:185–207

Mattis S (1976) Mental status examination for organic mental syndrome in the elderly patient. In: Bellack L, Karasu TB (eds) Geriatric psychiatry. Grune and Stratton, New York, pp 77–121

Melamed E, Mildworf B, Sharav T, Belenky L, Wertman E (1987) Regional cerebral blood flow in Down's syndrome. Ann Neurol 22:275–278

Neve RL, Rinch EA, Dawes LR (1988) Expression of the Alzheimer amyloid precursor gene transcripts in the human brain. Neuron 1:669–677

Rahmani Z, Blouin JL, Creau-Goldberg N, Watkins PC, Mattei JF, Poissonnier M, Prieur M, Chettouh Z, Nicole A, Aurias A, Sinet P-M, Delabar J-M (1989) Critical role of the D21S55 region on chromosome 21 in the pathogenesis of Down syndrome. Proc Natl Acad Sci USA 86:5958–5962

Risberg J (1980) Regional cerebral blood flow measurements by 133 Xe-inhalation: methodology and applications in neuropsychology and psychiatry. Brain Lang 9:9–34

Ropper AH, Williams RS (1980) Relationship between plaques, tangles, and dementia in Down syndrome. Neurology 30:639–644

Schapiro MB, Creasey H, Schwartz M, Haxby JV, White B, Moore A, Rapoport SI (1987a) Quantitative CT analysis of brain morphometry in adult Down's syndrome at different ages. Neurology 37:1424–1427

Schapiro MB, Grady CL, Kumar A, Herscovitch P, Haxby JV, Moore AM, White B, Friedland RP, Rapoport SI (1989a) Regional cerebral glucose metabolism is normal in young adults with Down syndrome. J Cereb Blood Flow Metab, in press

Schapiro MB, Haxby JV, Grady CL, Duara R, Schlageter NL, White B, Moore A, Sundaram M, Larson SM, Rapoport SI (1987b) Decline in cerebral glucose utilisation and cognitive function with aging in Down's syndrome. J Neurol Neurosurg Psychiat 50:766–774

Schapiro MB, Luxenberg JS, Kaye JA, Haxby JV, Friedland RP, Rapoport SI (1989b) Serial quantitative CT analysis of brain morphometrics in adult Down's syndrome at different ages. Neurology 39:1349–1353

Schwartz M, Creasey H, Grady CL, DeLeo JM, Frederickson HA, Cutler NR, Rapoport SI (1985) Computed tomographic analysis of brain morphometrics in 30 healthy men, aged 21 to 81 years. Ann Neurol 17:146–157

Schwartz M, Duara R, Haxby J, Grady C, White BJ, Kessler RM, Kay AD, Cutler NR, Rapoport SI (1983) Down's syndrome in adults: brain metabolism. Science 221:781–783

Solitare GB, Lamarche JB (1967) Brain weight in the adult mongol. J Ment Defic Res 11:79–84

St George-Hyslop PH, Tanzi RE, Polinsky RJ, Haines JL, Nee L, Watkins PC, Myers RH, Feldman RG, Pollen D, Drachman D, Growdon J, Bruni A, Foncin J-F, Salmon D, Frommelt P, Amaducci L, Sorbi S, Piacentini S, Stewart GD, Hobbs WJ, Conneally PM, Gusella JF (1987) The genetic defect causing familial Alzheimer's disease maps on chromosome 21. Science 235:885–890

Tanzi RE, Gusella JF, Watkins PC, Bruns GAP, St George-Hyslop P, Van Keuren ML, Patterson D, Pagan S, Kurnit DM, Neve RL (1987) Amyloid beta protein gene: cDNA, mRNA distribution, and genetic linkage near the Alzheimer locus. Science 235:880–884

Terman LM, Merrill MA (1973) Stanford-Binet Intelligence Scale: Manual for the Third Revision, Form L-M. Boston, Houghton-Mifflin

Wechsler DA (1955) Wechsler Adult Intelligence Scale. New York: Psychological Corporation

Wechsler D (1974) Wechsler Intelligence Scale for Children-Revised. Psychological Corporation, New York

Wisniewski KE, Wisniewski HM, Wen GY (1985) Occurrence of neuropathological changes and dementia of Alzheimer's disease in Down's syndrome. Ann Neurol 17:278–282

Yates CM, Simpson J, Gordon A, Maloney AFJ, Allison Y, Ritchie IM, Urquhart A (1983) Catecholamines and cholinergic enzymes in pre-senile and senile Alzheimer-type dementia and Down's syndrome. Brain Res 280:119–126

Cognitive Deficits and Local Metabolic Changes in Dementia of the Alzheimer Type

J. V. Haxby

Summary

Relations between neuropsychological and regional cerebral metabolic alterations were studied cross-sectionally and longitudinally in patients with dementia of the Alzheimer type and were compared to controls. Reductions in regional cerebral metabolism, measured in the resting state with positron emission tomography and [^{18}F]fluorodeoxyglucose, were greatest in the association cortices relative to the primary sensory and motor cortices and to the thalamus and basal ganglia. Individual patients demonstrated different patterns of association cortex metabolic reductions. Reductions in homologous right and left hemisphere association regions were often asymmetric. Parietal and frontal metabolic reductions were also often disproportionate relative to each other. Neuropsychological impairments in patients with dementia of the Alzheimer type were also selective and heterogeneous. Memory impairment was often the first symptom followed by impaired ability to maintain attention to complex or shifting sets. As the disease progressed, language and visuospatial functions became impaired. Whereas the memory impairment was usually global and severe, patterns of nonmemory impairments varied markedly from patient to patient. For example, some patients had disproportionately severe language impairments relative to milder visuospatial impairments and other patients demonstrated the opposite pattern. In patients with moderate dementia of the Alzheimer type, patterns of nonmemory impairments were related to the distribution of association cortex metabolic reductions. At initial evaluation, mildly impaired patients did not have significant nonmemory language and visuospatial impairments but did have significant neocortical metabolic reductions that were not correlated with neuropsychological test scores. After a mean of 2 years of longitudinal study, significant language and visuospatial impairments developed, and right-left metabolic asymmetries were significantly correlated with visuospatial-language discrepancies. These results suggest that neocortical metabolic abnormalities can be observed with positron emission tomography before associated impairments of neocortically mediated visuospatial and language functions are demonstrable.

Introduction

Alzheimer's disease is a progressive, degenerative brain disease whose principal clinical symptoms are disorders of memory, language and cognition. Other brain functions, such as simple sensory and motor function, are not impaired in patients with Alzheimer's disease or are impaired only in late stages after the dementia has become severe. The development of noninvasive methods to measure regional brain blood flow and metabolism has made it possible to examine relations between neuropsychological impairments and the regional distribution of disease-related alterations in blood flow and metabolism. In the Laboratory of Neurosciences, National Institute on Aging, we have been conducting a longitudinal study of patients with clinically diagnosed dementia of the Alzheimer type (DAT) for the past 7 years. At yearly intervals, patients are given positron emission tomography (PET) scans to measure regional cerebral metabolic rates for glucose (rCMRglc), computed tomography (CT) and MRI scans to examine brain structure, and an extensive battery of neuropsychological tests. In this paper, the major findings regarding the neuropsychological impairments associated with DAT and their relation to alterations in rCMRglc are reviewed. The emphasis in this review is on interindividual variations in the pattern of neuropsychological impairments and how these variations are related to patterns of rCMRglc reductions. These studies have helped to elucidate the neurobiological basis for disorders of language and visuospatial functions in DAT. Other prominent neuropsychological disorders of DAT, namely those of memory and attention, however, have not yet been related to regional brain alterations as measured with PET. The review concludes with a discussion of what the neurobiological basis of these disorders may be, why PET studies have heretofore not contributed to our understanding of these functions, and how future PET studies may be able to give us new insights in these areas.

Methods

Subjects

All patients with DAT met NINCDS-ADRDA diagnostic criteria for possible or probable Alzheimer's disease (McKhann et al. 1984) when studied initially. To study the full course of Alzheimer's disease, five patients were studied initially when they had an isolated memory impairment with no demonstrable impairments of nonmemory language or cognitive functions. Because dementia is a syndrome that by definition involves impairment of more than one area of cognitive function, these patients were not demented at the time of their first evaluation and met criteria for possible but not probable Alzheimer's disease. Subsequent evaluations of these patients demonstrated the development of nonmemory neuropsychological impairments in all five patients, and two have died with autopsy confirmation of Alzheimer's disease. Patients were divided into subgroups based on overall severity of dementia as measured by the Mini-Mental State Examination (Folstein et al. 1975). All patients in this study were normotensive and had no evidence of cardiovascular disease or any other current or past medical condition that could affect brain function. Control subjects for our study of DAT came from our longitudinal study of healthy aging. These subjects were similarly screened for optimal health and had no history of loss of mental abilities that could indicate an incipient dementia.

Neuropsychological Tests

An extensive battery of neuropsychological tests was administered to measure overall severity of dementia [Mattis Dementia Scale; Mattis 1976; Wechsler Adult Intelligence Scale (WAIS); Wechsler 1955], memory (Wechsler Memory Scale; Wechsler 1945), the ability to sustain attention to complex sets (Trailmaking; Reitan 1958; Stroop Color Word; Golden 1978), planning (Porteus Mazes; Porteus 1965), language (syntax comprehension; Whitehouse in Haxby et al. 1985; Controlled Word Association; Benton 1973), and visuospatial function (Extended Range Drawing; Haxby et al. 1985; Block tapping span; Milner 1971).

Positron Emission Tomography

Regional cerebral metabolic rates for glucose (rCMRglc) were measured in the resting state (eyes covered, ears plugged) with PET and [^{18}F]2-fluoro-2-D-deoxyglucose (FDG) as described elsewhere (Duara et al. 1986; Haxby et al. 1985). Scanning was accomplished with an ECAT-II scanner (ORTEC, Life Sciences, Oak Ridge, TN) which has an in-plane resolution of 1.7 cm full width at half maximum. For the analyses reviewed here, rCMRglc in 14 neocortical regions (7/hemisphere) of interest were calculated. These regions were the prefrontal, premotor, orbitofrontal, sensorimotor, parietal association, lateral temporal and occipital cortices.

Neuropsychological and Metabolic Pattern Indices

To examine patterns of neuropsychological impairments and rCMRglc reductions in patients with DAT, indices that contrast performance on selected pairs of tests or contrast metabolic rates in selected pairs of regions were calculated. Neuropsychological discrepancies were calculated as the difference between ranked scores on most tests because of the uncertain scaling properties. For factor deviation quotients (DQ) calculated from the WAIS, which have well-controlled scaling properties, the difference betweeen scores was used. Right-left rCMRglc asymmetries were calculated as $2(R - L)/(R + L)$, where R and L refer to rCMRglc values in homologous right and left hemisphere regions. Parietal-frontal rCMRglc discrepancies were calculated as ratios.

Neuropsychological Impairments in DAT

Patients with mild DAT had selective patterns of neuropsychological impairments (Table 1). The ability to commit new information to long-term memory was consistently and globally impaired in these patients. Nonmemory language and visuospatial functions were not significantly impaired relative to controls. As mentioned above, five patients had significant impairments, defined as a test score more than 2 SD below the control mean, on only memory tests when they were first tested. Nonetheless, as a group, the ten patients with mild DAT differed significantly from controls on tests of complex attention and planning, indicating that these functions are the next, after memory, to demonstrate impairment in

Table 1. Neuropsychological test scores for controls and patients with mild and moderate dementia of the Alzheimer type (DAT). Score on the Mini-Mental State Examination (Folstein et al. 1976) was used to define severity groups with scores over 21 denoting mild impairment and scores between 11 and 21 denoting moderate impairment[a]

Test	Controls ($N = 19-29$)	Mild DAT[b] ($N = 10$)	Moderate DAT ($N = 14$)
Summary measures			
Mattis dementia scale	142 ± 2	132 ± 6*	110 ± 17***
WAIS			
Full-scale IQ	125 ± 10	117 ± 8	90 ± 19***
Deviation quotients (DQ)			
Verbal comprehension	129 ± 10	122 ± 9	99 ± 19***
Memory and distractibility	116 ± 14	114 ± 9	90 ± 16***
Perceptual organization	119 ± 13	108 ± 13	83 ± 25***
Memory			
Wechsler memory scale			
Immediate story recall	22 ± 5	11 ± 5**	5 ± 3***
Immediate visual recall	10 ± 3	6 ± 5**	1.4 ± 1.8***
Delayed story recall	17 ± 5	2.6 ± 3.7***	0.7 ± 1.1***
Delayed visual recall	7 ± 3	0.8 ± 1.1***	0.3 ± 0.7***
Attention and planning			
Trailmaking (trail A, s)	40 ± 17	54 ± 30	153 ± 98***
Trailmaking (trail B, s)	84 ± 38	202 ± 159**	434 ± 134***
Stroop color word	37 ± 9	24 ± 8**	12 ± 8***
Porteus mazes (test age)	15.4 ± 1.5	12.5 ± 3.9*	7.5 ± 3.7
Language			
Syntax comprehension	24 ± 3	23 ± 2	17 ± 5***
Controlled word association	42 ± 15	31 ± 8	23 ± 12***
Visuospatial			
Extended range drawing	21 ± 2	19 ± 4	13 ± 5***
Block tapping span	29 ± 6	25 ± 4	19 ± 7***

[a] From Haxby et al. (1988)
[b] Differs from controls (probabilities corrected for three comparisons): * $p < 0.05$, ** $p < 0.01$, *** $p < 0.001$

early DAT. These tests were also the first to show significant impairments in a case-by-case longitudinal analysis of the patients with isolated memory impairment initially (Grady et al. 1988).

In contrast to the patients with mild DAT, patients with moderate DAT differed significantly from controls on all neuropsychological tests. In individual patients, however, nonmemory language and cognitive functions were not uniformly impaired. For example, some patients had disproportionately severe impairment of language function relative to milder impairment of visuospatial construction, whereas other patients had the opposite pattern. The pattern of other nonmemory neuropsychological impairments, such as calculations, attention to simple tasks, and immediate visuospatial memory, also varied considerably among the patients with moderate DAT. These variations in the pattern of neuropsychological impairments suggested variably distributed alterations in neocortical function, which could be examined directly with PET studies of resting rCMRglc.

Neocortical Metabolic Patterns in DAT

The largest reductions of rCMRglc in patients with Alzheimer's disease are consistently found in the association areas of the neocortex (Haxby et al. 1985, 1986, 1988; Duara et al. 1986). By contrast, the primary sensorimotor cortices, primary visual cortices, cerebellum, thalamus, caudate and lenticular nuclei tend to demonstrate relative sparing of resting state rCMRglc. The association cortices demonstrate selective and significant alterations even in patients with very early DAT, including those patients with only isolated memory impairment (Haxby et al. 1986, 1988; Grady et al. 1988). PET studies, therefore, suggest that Alzheimer's disease selectively affects the association systems of the brain in the very early stages.

The parietal association cortex usually demonstrates the greatest metabolic abnormalities, especially in earlier stages of DAT, but the pattern of association cortex metabolic reductions varies considerably among patients. This heterogeneity in the cerebral topography of disease-related alterations is evident as asymmetric reductions in homologous right and left hemisphere regions (Fig. 1) and as discrepant reductions in the parietal and frontal association cortices (Fig. 2). Right-left asymmetries of rCMRglc have increased variances in patients with Alzheimer's disease as compared to controls (Haxby et al. 1985, 1986; Duara et al. 1986; Friedland et al. 1985; McGeer et al. 1986). Equivalent numbers of patients have left-sided and right-sided asymmetries, and approximately one-third of patients with DAT have symmetric rCMRglc values in all the association cortices. The frontal, parietal and temporal association cortices all demonstrate significantly increased asymmetry at all stages of DAT, indicating that all association cortices are affected throughout the course of DAT. Primary sensorimotor and occipital cortex rCMRglc values, however, are not more asymmetric in patients with DAT than in controls, again demonstrating the relative sparing of these areas.

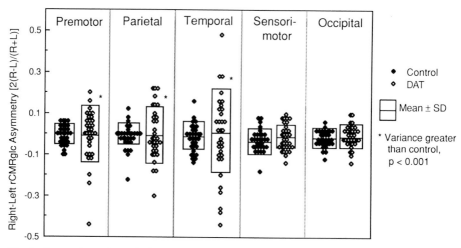

Fig. 1. Scatterplots of association cortex and primary cortex right-left metabolic asymmetries in 33 patients with Alzheimer's disease and 31 controls

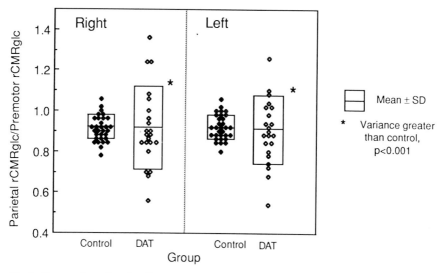

Fig. 2. Scatterplots of parietal/premotor metabolic ratios for controls ($N = 31$) and patients with moderate and severe DAT ($N = 22$). (Haxby et al. 1988)

The ratio of parietal association cortex to premotor cortex rCMRglc also has increased variance in patients with DAT relative to controls (Fig. 2; Haxby et al. 1988). Some patients have disproportionate reductions of premotor rCMRglc, whereas others have disproportionate parietal metabolic reductions. These results demonstrate that the association cortical regions most affected in DAT vary significantly among individual patients. This topographical heterogeneity could be the basis for the variable patterns of nonmemory language and cognitive impairments noted in moderately demented patients.

Relations Between Cognitive and Metabolic Patterns

In moderately demented patients with DAT, the neuropsychological discrepancy between language and visuospatial impairments was consistently and significantly correlated with right-left metabolic asymmetries (Fig. 3, Table 2; Haxby et al. 1985, 1986, 1987). These relations were all in the expected direction. Disproportionate left-sided hypometabolism was associated with disproportionate language impairment, whereas disproportionate right-sided hypometabolism was associated with visuospatial impairment. Similarly, parietal-frontal metabolic ratios were significantly correlated with neuropsychological discrepancies in moderately demented patients (Fig. 4), such that disproportionate frontal hypometabolism was associated with impairments of verbal fluency and simple attention (trail A), and disproportionate parietal hypometabolism was associated with impairments of verbal comprehension, calculations, visuospatial construction and immediate visuospatial memory span (Haxby et al. 1988).

These findings clearly demonstrated that interindividual differences in the pattern of nonmemory language and cognitive impairments in patients with moderate DAT were attributable to differences in the topographical distribution of disease-related alterations in regional brain function. Patients with mild DAT, on the other hand, did not demonstrate significant impairments of these nonmemory neuropsychological functions, yet they demonstrated the same variably distributed association cortex metabolic reductions. Moreover, their patterns of nonmemory language and cognitive test scores were uncorrelated with right-left rCMRglc asymmetries (Table 2; Haxby et al. 1986) and parietal-frontal rCMRglc ratios (Haxby et al. 1988). After a mean follow-up period of 24 months (range, 13–40 months), however, these patients had developed significant impairments of nonmemory visuospatial and language functions, and the discrepancies between visu-

Table 2. Correlations between right-left metabolic asymmetries and visuospatial-verbal discrepancies in patients with moderate DAT and in patients with mild DAT at initial and follow-up evaluations. Mean follow-up duration was 24 months (range, 14–40 months)[a]

Neuropsychological discrepancy index	rCMRglc Asymmetry	Controls (N=12)	Moderate DAT (N=12)	Mild DAT (N=10)	
				Initial	Follow-up
Syntax comprehension[b] versus drawing	Frontal	−0.30	0.71**	−0.01	0.66*
	Parietal	−0.11	0.73**	−0.20	0.46
	Temporal	−0.08	0.49	0.01	0.44
WAIS PDQ-MDQ	Frontal	0.08	0.59*	−0.08	0.57
	Parietal	0.12	0.76**	−0.06	0.47
	Temporal	−0.07	0.58*	0.05	0.42
WAIS PDQ-VDQ	Frontal	−0.14	0.45	−0.20	0.66*
	Parietal	−0.15	0.49	−0.15	0.58
	Temporal	0.29	0.35	−0.10	0.61

[a] From Haxby et al. (1987)
[b] Symbols: * $p<0.05$; ** $p<0.01$

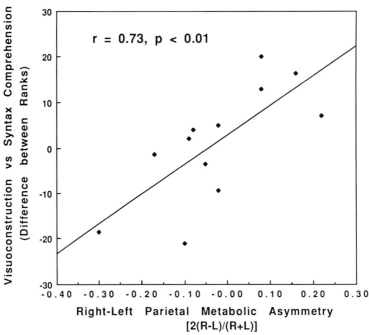

Fig. 3. Scatterplot of the relation between parietal right-left metabolic asymmetry and visuospatial-verbal neuropsychological discrepancy in 12 patients with moderate DAT. (Haxby et al. 1986, 1987)

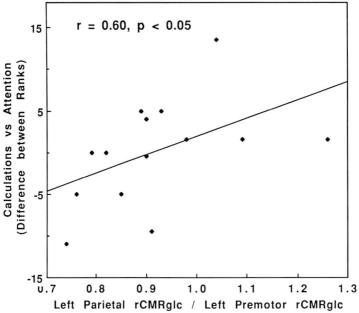

Fig. 4. Scatterplot of the relation between left parietal/premotor metabolic ratio and the neuropsychological discrepancy between ability to attend to a simple set and calculations in 14 patients with moderate DAT. (Haxby et al. 1988)

ospatial and language impairments were correlated in the expected direction with right-left metabolic asymmetries (Table 2; Haxby et al. 1987). Over this same interval, the direction and magnitude of right-left metabolic asymmetries were remarkably stable (Grady et al. 1986). These results indicate that neocortical metabolic abnormalities can be observed with PET before their neuropsychological consequences are demonstrable with standardized neuropsychological tests.

It is important to emphasize that abnormal rCMRglc patterns have not been demonstrated in preclinical stages of DAT. Although five of our patients were not demented when first tested, they had marked and easily demonstrated memory impairment. One of these patients also had a normal PET scan initially and went on to develop rCMRglc abnormalities before his language and visuospatial functions worsened (Grady et al. 1988), suggesting that memory impairment precedes neocortical metabolic abnormalities in DAT.

It is also important to note that the relation of cerebral metabolic abnormalities to impairment of attention to complex or shifting sets is not clear. Thus, although PET studies have elucidated the neurobiological basis of cognitive impairments associated with intermediate stages of DAT, they have provided little information about the neurobiological basis for the neuropsychological symptoms of very early DAT. Because opportunities for neuropathological study of very early DAT are exceedingly scarce, further understanding in this area will depend on in vivo study methods such as PET.

Normal recent memory depends on interaction between neocortical regions and non-neocortical memory structures such as the hippocampus, amygdala and medial thalamus. Mishkin has proposed that memory is encoded in the neocortical regions that initially processed the information to be remembered (Mishkin and Appenzeller 1987). Interaction with the non-neocortical memory structures enables the changes necessary to encode the memory. Given this basis for normal memory, there are several possible causes for memory impairment in early DAT. Neuropathological damage to the hippocampus and amygdala is consistently severe in Alzheimer's disease (Ball 1976) and is perhaps the most likely cause for memory impairment. Loss of cells in the entorhinal cortex that serve as relays between neocortex and hippocampus (Hyman et al. 1986), or loss of neocortical pyramidal cells that project to memory structures (see Morrison et al., this volume), may also impair memory by disrupting interactions between neocortex and memory structures. Finally, cytoskeletal abnormalities in neocortical neurons could impair formation of structural changes that may underlie the encoding of new memories. The memory impairment in DAT, therefore, may be due to dysfunction in non-neocortical structures too small to study with low-resolution PET, to impaired interaction between brain structures or to neocortical dysfunction.

Normal attentional function also involves interactions between widely dispersed brain structures in neocortex, allocortex and brainstem (Mesulam 1981). Both the memory and attentional impairments associated with very early DAT, therefore, may be related to impaired interaction between brain regions or to impairment to the regions themselves. The special vulnerability of these functions may be related to the selective involvement of neocortical cell groups whose axons form long cortico-cortical projections (see Morrison et al., this volume). A method for examining inter-regional functional associations with PET has been developed by Horwitz et al. (1987) that may help elucidate the extent to which the early neuropsychological impairments in DAT are attributable to disrupted communication between brain regions. This method uses interregional correlations as indices of the strength of the functional association between brain regions. By determining the functional associations that become active during memory formation or directing attention, diminution of these associations in patients with DAT can be studied and related to the severity of their neuropsychological impairments.

Studies of resting state regional cerebral metabolism in patients with DAT have shown that the disease selectively involves the association neocortices and that the distribution of association cortex metabolic alterations varies markedly among patients. These interindividual variations in the cerebral topography of Alzheimer's disease underlie interindividual variations in the pattern of nonmemory language and visuospatial impairments that are evident in patients with moderate dementia. In earlier stages of DAT, neocortical metabolic abnormalities are observed before neocortically mediated language and visuospatial impairments are demonstrable. PET studies have yet to elucidate the neurobiological basis for earlier neuropsychological impairments of memory and complex attention. Better PET methods, such as high-resolution tomographs and sophisticated multivariate procedures for examining patterns of connectivity, may provide the analytic tools necessary for further understanding about the earliest alterations in brain function that have neuropsychological consequences in Alzheimer's disease.

References

Ball MJ (1976) Neurofibrillary tangles and the pathogenesis of dementia: a quantitative study. Neuropathol Appl Neurobiol 2:395–410

Benton AL (1973) The measurement of aphasic disorders. In: Velasquez AC (ed) Aspectos Patologicos del Langage. Centro Neuropsicologico, Lima, Peru

Duara R, Grady CL, Haxby JV, Sundaram M, Cutler NR, Heston L, Morre A, Schlageter NL, Larson S, Rapoport SI (1986) Positron emission tomography in Alzheimer's disease. Neurology 36:879–887

Folstein MF, Folstein SE, McHugh PR (1975) 'Mini-Mental State': a practical method for grading the mental state of patients for the clinician. J Psychiat Res 12:189–198

Friedland RP, Budinger TF, Koss E, Ober BA (1985) Alzheimer's disease: anterior-posterior and lateral hemispheric alterations in cortical glucose utilization. Neurosci Lett 53:235–240

Golden CJ (1978) The Stroop color and word test: a manual for clinical and experimental uses. Stoelting, Chicago

Grady CL, Haxby JV, Schlageter NL, Berg G, Rapoport SI (1986) Stability of metabolic and neuropsychological asymmetries in dementia of the Alzheimer type. Neurology 36:1390–1392

Grady CL, Haxby JV, Horwitz B, Sundaram M, Berg G, Schapiro M, Friedland RP, Rapoport SI (1988) A longitudinal study of the early neuropsychological and cerebral metabolic changes in dementia of the Alzheimer type. J Clin Exp Neuropsychol 10:576–596

Haxby JV, Duara R, Grady CL, Cutler NR, Rapoport SI (1985) Relations between neuropsychological and cerebral metabolic asymmetries in early Alzheimer's disease. J Cereb Blood Flow Metabol 5:193–200

Haxby JV, Grady CL, Duara R, Schlageter NL, Berg G, Rapoport SI (1986) Neocortical metabolic abnormalities precede non-memory cognitive deficits in early Alzheimer-type dementia. Arch Neurol 43:882–885

Haxby JV, Grady CL, Friedland RP, Rapoport SI (1987) Neocortical metabolic abnormalities precede nonmemory cognitive impairments in early dementia of the Alzheimer type: longitudinal confirmation. J Neural Transm 24[Suppl]:49–51

Haxby JV, Grady CL, Koss E, Horwitz B, Schapiro M, Friedland RP, Rapoport SI (1988) Heterogeneous anterior-posterior metabolic patterns in Alzheimer's type dementia. Neurology 38:1853–1863

Horwitz B, Grady CL, Schlageter NL, Duara R, Rapoport SI (1987) Intercorrelations of regional cerebral glucose metabolic rates in Alzheimer's disease. Brain Res 407:294–306

Hyman BT, Van Hoesen GW, Kromer LJ, Damasio AR (1986) Perforant pathway changes and the memory impairment in Alzheimer's disese. Ann Neurol 20:472–481

Mattis S (1976) Mental status examination for organic mental syndrome in the elderly patient. In: Bellack L, Karasu TB (eds) Geriatric psychiatry, Grune & Stratton, New York, pp 77–121

McGeer PL, Kamo H, Harrop R, Li DKB, Tuokko H, McGeer EG, Adam MJ, Ammann W, Beattie BL, Calne DB, Martin WBW, Pate BD, Rogers JG, Ruth TJ, Sayre CI, Stoessl AJ (1986) Positron emission tomography in patients with clinically diagnosed Alzheimer's disease. Can Med Assoc J 134:597–607

McKhann G, Drachman D, Folstein M, Katzman R, Price D, Stadlan EM (1984) Clinical diagnosis of Alzheimer's disease: report of the NINCDS-ADRDA Work Group under the auspices of Department of Health and Human Services Task Force on Alzheimer's Disease. Neurology 34:939–944

Mesulam MM (1981) A cortical network for directed attention and unilateral neglect. Ann Neurol 10:309–325

Milner B (1971) Interhemispheric difference in the localization of psychological process in man. Br Med Bull 27:272–277

Mishkin M, Appenzeller T (1987) The anatomy of memory. Sci Am 256:80–89

Porteus SD (1965) Porteus Maze Test: fifty years application. Pacific Books, Palo Alto

Reitan RM (1958) Validity of the trail making test as an indicator of organic brain damage. Percept Mot Skills 8:271–276

Wechsler DA (1945) A standardized memory scale for clinical use. J Psychol 19:87–95

Wechsler DA (1955) Wechsler Adult Intelligence Scale. Psychological Corporation, New York

Patterns of Cerebral Metabolism in Degenerative Dementia

M. N. Rossor, P. J. Tyrrell, and R. S. J. Frackowiak

Summary

Alzheimer's disease is the commonest cause of primary degenerative dementia and classically presents with early memory disturbance and subsequent impairment of language and visuospatial functions. Characteristically positron emission tomography (PET) scanning reveals posterior biparietal and bitemporal hypometabolism. Increasingly, clinical subtypes of Alzheimer's disease are being recognized, although it is not yet clear whether these represent biological distinctions. The most clearly defined is the distinction between familial and sporadic cases. PET studies to date, however, reveal no obvious differences. Similarly, both early- and late-onset cases may demonstrate posterior biparietal hypometabolism. A further distinction is that drawn between rigid and non-rigid cases. It has been argued that Parkinsonian features are a frequent finding in Alzheimer's disease and may be due to coincidental Lewy body formation. We have examined 20 patients for the presence of extrapyramidal features and confirm that rigidity may be demonstrated in a number of these cases, but this is not always accompanied by the bradykinesia that is characteristic of Parkinson's disease. In addition, [^{18}F]fluorodopa uptake studied with PET shows no significant differences between rigid and non-rigid Alzheimer's patients, or between patients and healthy controls, in contrast to the marked reduction in putamen uptake in Parkinson's disease. These findings suggest that extranigral factors contribute to the rigidity in this group. In addition to Alzheimer's disease, non-Alzheimer primary degenerative dementias are being increasingly recognized. These include the frontal lobe dementias and focal cortical degenerations, such as primary progressive dysphasia, which may progress to a late generalized cognitive impairment. PET scanning in these groups reveals neither diffuse frontal lobe hypometabolism in the frontal lobe dementia group or focal hypometabolism in the left temporal lobe in patients with primary progressive dysphasia.

Introduction

Dementia is commonly recognized in the elderly, with prevalence figures ranging between 5% and 20% of those aged above 65 and 80 years, respectively. Prospective autopsy studies indicate that about 50% of elderly dementia cases will be due to Alzheimer's disease, with a further 20%–25% being due to Alzheimer's disease in combination with vascular disease. The characteristic features of senile plaques, neurofibrillary tangles and neuronal cell loss within the cerebral cortex are found predominantly within association areas. This anatomical distribution of the histopathology is reflected in the pattern of hypometabolism that may be observed in vivo using PET, which is believed to reflect cell loss and disintegration. Posterior biparietal and bitemporal hypometabolism, demonstrated using 15-oxygen (Frackowiak et al. 1981) to determine regional $CMRO_2$, is matched by an equivalent fall in cerebral blood flow and maintenance of normal oxygen extraction (OER). The posterior biparietal and bitemporal hypometabolism, with late bifrontal hypometabolism in more severe cases, is now seen as a characteristic feature of Alzheimer's disease, and has been subsequently confirmed as reduced glucose metabolism using [^{18}F]fluorodeoxyglucose (Friedland et al. 1983). There is an overall association between the severity of dementia and the degree of hypometabolism, although within this overall pattern associations have been observed between specific patterns of neuropsychological deficit and anterior-posterior and left-right asymmetries of hypometabolism (Frackowiak et al. 1981; Foster et al. 1983; Duara et al. 1986). The overall pattern of hypometabolism, together with asymmetries within an individual patient, is relatively stable over time (Jagust et al. 1988).

Posterior biparietal and bitemporal hypometabolism is a characteristic feature of clinically diagnosed cases of Alzheimer's disease and, if observed, may help to support the diagnosis. However, there is a general paucity of reported cases which have been followed to autopsy to assess the specificity of this pattern; a similar pattern of hypometabolism, for example, has been observed in Creutzfeldt-Jakob disease (Friedland et al. 1984). Moreover, it is not known whether histologically established cases of Alzheimer's disease might show alternative patterns of hypometabolism, or to what extent patterns of metabolism might differ between the clinical subtypes of Alzheimer's disease.

Positron Emission Scanning in Subtypes of Alzheimer's Disease

Alzheimer's disease was originally considered a rare disorder occurring in the presenium, and a distinction was thus drawn between presenile dementia of the Alzheimer type and senile dementia. With the histological studies in the 1960s this distinction was no longer drawn, and current usage covers all cases of dementia associated with the characteristic histopathological change. Recently, however, a distinction has again been drawn between early- and late-onset cases of Alzheimer's disease which may differ clinically, with a higher prevalence of language disturbance in early-onset cases (Seltzer and Sherwin 1983). More severe histopathological change in the early-onset patients and a more widespread neurochemical deficit (Rossor et al. 1984) have been reported. Similarly more prominent metabolic asymmetries have been observed with lower left parietal metabolism in the early-onset (<65 years of age) patient compared with later onset (>65 years of age) cases (Grady et al. 1987; Small et al. 1989).

It is not clear whether the age groups reflect a true nosological distinction or merely a biological continuum. A more secure distinction can be made with the subgroup of patients with familial Alzheimer's disease with an autosomal dominant pattern of inheritance. Originally this form was thought to be a rarity, but it has been suggested that as many as 60% of cases may be familial (Heyman et al. 1984). The hereditary pattern may not be apparent due to the fact that family members frequently die from unrelated causes before the phenotypic expression of a familial Alzheimer's disease gene. The few published cases of familial Alzheimer's disease which have been scanned using [^{18}F]fluorodeoxyglucose also indicate a pattern of posterior biparietal hypometabolism (Polinksy et al. 1987; Cutler et al. 1985).

Clinical subgroups have also been suggested on the basis of clinical features such as the cognitive profile, presence of myoclonus or the presence of extrapyramidal features. Extrapyramidal abnormalities have been reported in as many as 90% of patients with Alzheimer's disease, with rigidity being the predominant abnormality found on examination (Molsa et al. 1984; Mayeux et al. 1985; Chui et al. 1985). It has been suggested that the presence of extrapyramidal features is due to the coexistence of Lewy body pathology in the substantia nigra and a consequent presynaptic dopamine deficit (Ditter and Mirra 1987). However, in a recent prospective study, 36% of patients were found to have extrapyramidal features, but these were not necesarily associated with the presence of Lewy body pathology at autopsy. Of the cases examined at autopsy, approximately 50% were found to have nigral Lewy body pathology but its absence in other cases, and in some entirely normal nigral histology, argues for extranigral components in the pathophysiology of rigidity (Morris et al. 1989). In addition, the lack of response to levodopa argues against a simple presynaptic dopamine deficit (Duret et al. 1989).

We have examined 20 patients (mean age, 59.1 ± 8.5 years; range 40–74 years) with a clinical diagnosis of Alzheimer's disease who fulfilled the NINCDS clinical criteria (McKhann et al. 1984). A subgroup of 15 patients was scanned with [^{18}F]fluorodopa as described previously (Leenders et al. 1986). None of these patients was on neuroleptic medication. Nine of 15 patients were found to have rigidity on examination and 6 were considered to have no motor abnormality. Comparisons were made betweeen these two groups and with seven normal subjects (mean age, 57.1 ± 9.7 years; range 43–67 years). The K_i values (the influx constants calculated using the multiple time graphic analysis approach; Patlak and Blasberg 1985) for uptake of [^{18}F]flurodopa are shown in Table 1.

There was no statistically significant difference between the mean K_i for putamen and caudate either between the non-rigid and rigid Alzheimer cases or by comparison with the control group. This is in contrast to the 60% reduction in K_i for fluorodopa uptake into the putamen reported in Parkinson's disease (Leenders et al. 1986). The proportion of Alzheimer patients (60%) who were found clinically to have extrapyramidal features is similar to previous observations (Molsa et al. 1984; Mayeux et al. 1985; Chui et al. 1985); however, the clinical features were those of rigidity without the bradykinesia which is a prominent feature of Parkinson's disease. Moreover, not only were there no clinical features of bradykinesia but no symptoms such as difficulty arising from a chair on

Table 1. Mean K_i values for caudate and putamen for the normal subjects and the two patient groups

	K_i caudate		K_i putamen	
	Mean	SD	Mean	SD
Normal	0.0104	0.0005	0.0112	0.0010
Non-rigid DAT	0.0119	0.0018	0.0109	0.0020
Rigid DAT	0.0119	0.0016	0.0097	0.0015

SD, standard deviation; DAT, dementia of Alzheimer type

turning over in bed were reported by the patient (Tyrrell and Rossor 1989 a). The rigidity was of the "cogwheeling" type, which was increased by contralateral reinforcement; however, three patients were found to have non-cogwheeling rigidity, which was unchanged by contralateral reinforcement but which altered in response to the variations in force and amplitude of the applied stimulus. This was considered to be more similar to the rigidity referred to as gegenhalten, which might relate to upper limb dyspraxia rather than to extrapyramidal disease (Tyrrell and Rossor 1988).

Focal Cortical Degenerations

Dementia is defined as cognitive impairment affecting multiple domains, but within this global impairment focal neuropsychological deficits can be discerned which show association with regional hypometabolism (Foster et al. 1983; Haxby et al. 1985). Alzheimer's disease may, however, present focally, for example with dysphasia (Kirshner et al. 1984). In these patients a global dementia occurs relatively early, but in some patients a focal neuropsychological deficit on the basis of focal degeneration may persist for a long time before more widespread cognitive impairment supervenes. The most widely recognized syndrome is that of slowly progressive dysphasis due to left perisylvian atrophy (Mesulam 1982; Poeck and Luzzati 1988). Patients with occipital atrophy presenting with visual agnosia have also been described (Benson et al. 1988), but this may be an early presentation of Alzheimer's disease. We have examined the pattern of regional cerebral oxygen metabolism using oxygen-15 in a variety of focal cortical degenerations.

Primary Progressive Dysphasia

We examined six patients with progressive dysphasia (age 44–73 years) with a variable length of history from 2–6 years and with a variable severity of dysphasia (Tyrrell et al. 1989a). The least severely affected patient had a 4-year history of difficulty with remembering certain low frequency words and was found to have an isolated naming deficit which was apparent only on the graded difficulty naming test (McKenna and Warrington 1983), with satisfactory performance of the Oldfield naming test. He had a verbal IQ score of 129, performance IQ of 121 and a premorbid estimate on the National Adult Reading Test (NART) of 121. The most severely affected patient was tested initially after a 1-year history of language disturbance, when he was found to have a nominal dysphasia with a verbal IQ of 85 and a performance IQ of 110. He suffered progressive deterioration in language function and, at the time of scanning, there was no meaningful speech or comprehension, which included a failure to understand simple gestures. Despite this profound language deficit he had been driving a car without getting lost and carrying out domestic tasks. Moreover, although the language deficit precluded formal neuropsychological testing, when he was finally able to understand what was required he scored at the 70th percentile on the colour matrices, indicating that his non-verbal reasoning was relatively intact.

Oxygen-15 steady-state PET scans were used to obtain regional values for $CMRO_2$. All cases revealed left-right asymmetries in the temporal lobe, with a maximal area of hypometabolism anteriorly in the superior temporal gyrus on the left, with one single exception, in which the maximal area of hypometabolism was found in the postfrontal gyrus on the left, adjacent to the Sylvian fissure. The more severe cases had the more widespread areas of hypometabolism and, interestingly, the most severe patient had widespread left hemisphere hypometabolism and, in addition, a small area of hypometabolism in the anterior right temporal lobe. These patients did not have the pattern of posterior biparietal hypometabolism, and the less severe cases were similar to the two reported cases which were scanned using [18F]fluorodeoxyglucose (Chawluk et al. 1986).

The underlying histopathology in these cases is unknown. Some patients presenting with dysphasia are found to have Alzheimer histopathology. Two cases of primary progressive dysphasia which were followed to autopsy were found to have a non-specific spongiform degeneration in the left temporal lobe (Kirshner et al. 1987). Other cases may be focal presentations of Pick's disease or frontal lobe dementias (Gustafson 1987; Neary et al. 1988). Bifrontal hypometabolism has been reported using [18F]fluorodeoxyglucose scanning in a case of Pick's disease which correlated with the extent of gliosis at autopsy (Kamo et al. 1987) but did not show the striking asymmetry found in these cases. A pattern of reduced bifrontal cerebral blood flow has also been demonstrated by single photon emission computer tomography using HMPAO (Neary et al. 1988).

The nature of the predilection for the left temporal lobe is unclear. The most severe case in this series showed a small area of hypometabolism in the anterior right temporal lobe. This raises the possibility of a pathogenic agent progressing by reciprocal transcallosal connections. Alternatively, the anterior temporal lobes may show regional selective vulnerability, but if so it is not clear why the left temporal lobe should show greater vulnerability than the right. There are minor neurochemical differences reported, such as in choline acetyltransferase activity (Sorbi et al. 1984), and there are observed differences in cytoarchitectural detail. Alternatively, the apparent predilection of the left temporal lobe may reflect the clinical eloquence of lesions at this site. There have been no reported cases of selective right temporal lobe degeneration, although we have scanned one patient who might represent such an example (Tyrrell et al. 1989 b). A 79-year-old man presented with a 12-year progressive history of prosopagnosia such that he was unable to recognize members of his own family. He had a more recent history of mild naming difficulty. He was found to have a verbal IQ of 117 and a performance IQ of 101 on the Wechsler Adult Intelligence Scale. His performance was satisfactory on a wide range of cognitive tests including verbal comprehension and memory. However, his visuoperceptual and visual memory functions were weak, scoring less than the 5th percentile on unusual views and recognition memory of faces, despite adequate performance on shape discrimination and detection. However, the most profound deficit was in his ability to recognize familiar faces, although he was able to perform satisfactorily on the verbal version of the task (Warrington and McCarthy 1988). The naming difficulty that the patient experienced was confirmed with poor performance on the graded naming task, despite adequate performance on the Oldfield picture naming test. PET scanning with oxygen-15 revealed a marked reduction of oxygen metabolism in the anterior right temporal lobe and a less severe area of hypometabolism in the left anterior temporal lobe. Regional oxygen metabolism was normal in the occipital, parietal and frontal cortices.

Patients with occipital lobe atrophy present with progressive visual impairment resulting in cortical blindness (Benson et al. 1988). Two patients who have been scanned revealed bilateral occipital hypometabolism (Tyrrell et al. 1989 b), which projected forward into the posterior parietal and posterior temporal lobes, showing greater similarity to the pattern found in Alzheimer's disease (Frackowiak et al. 1982) than the more focal deficits found in patients with progressive dysphasia.

Conclusion

Positron emission tomography with oxygen-15 has proven to be a powerful technique for demonstrating regions of hypometabolism, and, thus, presumed areas of cellular pathology, which may not be apparent on the structural images obtained with magnetic resonance imaging and computer tomography scanning. Alzheimer's disease may present with a focal neuropsychological deficit but dementia intervenes early; this is quite unlike the focal cortical degenerations, which may have a history of a progressive neuropsychological deficit for more than 10 years before a global dementia intervenes. The areas of hypometabolism reflect the specificity of the neuropsychological deficit and raise intriguing questions of regional selective vulnerability within the cerebral cortex. These cases do not show the posterior biparietal hypometabolism which is found in Alzheimer's disease, although the precise specificity and sensitivity of this pattern have still to be determined in prospective autopsy studies. However, within the subgroups of Alzheimer's disease studied, biparietal hypometabolism remains a consistent feature. The development of ligands for exploring defined neurotransmitter systems opens new avenues for the determination of selective vulnerability in Alzheimer's disease. The preserved fluorodopa uptake in Alzheimer patients with and without rigidity argues for extranigral factors in the pathophysiology of rigidity and provides further evidence of the selective vulnerability, with sparing of the dopamine system in the majority of patients. With the availability of further ligands in the future, the associations made between focal neuropsychological deficits and regional metabolism can be extended to the relationship of defined neurotransmitter systems within these areas to specific cognitive functions.

Acknowledgements. We are grateful to Prof. E. K. Warrington and Dr. F. Clegs for neuropsychological assessment and to the staff of the Chemistry, Physics and Engineering sections of the MRC Cyclotron Unit. The studies reported here were supported by a project grant from the Medical Research Council.

References

Benson DF, Davis RJ, Snyder BD (1988) Posterior cortical atrophy. Arch Neurol 33:789–793

Chawluk JB, Mesulam M-M, Hurtig H, Kushner M, Weintraub S, Saykin A (1986) Slowly progressive aphasia without generalised dementia: studies with positron emission tomography. Ann Neurol 19:68–74

Chui HC, Teng EL, Henderson V, Moy AC (1985) Clinical subtypes of dementia of the Alzheimer type. Neurology 35:1544–1550

Cutler NR, Haxby JV, Duara R, et al. (1985) Brain metabolism as measured with positron emission tomography: serial assessments in a patient with familial Alzheimer's disease. Neurology 35:1556–1561

Ditter SM, Mirra SS (1987) Neuropathologic and clinical features of Parkinson's disease in Alzheimer's disease patients. Neurology 37:754–760

Duara R, Grady C, Haxby J, Sundason M, Cutler NR, Heston L, Moore A, Schlageter N, Larson S, Rapoport SI (1986) Positron emission tomography in Alzheimer's disease. Neurology 36:879–887

Duret M, Goldman S, Messina D, Hildebrand J (1989) Effects of L-dopa on dementia related rigidity. Acta Neurol Scand, in press

Foster NL, Chase TN, Fedio P, Patronas NJ, Brooks RA, Di Chiro G (1983) Alzheimer's disease: focal cortical changes shown by positron emission tomography. Neurology 33:961–965

Frackowiak RSJ, Pozzilli C, Legg NJ, Du Boulay GH, Marshall J, Jones T (1981) Regional cerebral oxygen supply and utilisation in dementia. A clinical and physiological study with oxygen-15 and positron tomography. Brain 104:753–778

Friedland RP, Budinger TS, Ganz E, Yano Y, Mathis CA, Koss B, Ober BA, Heusman RH, Derenzo SE (1983) Regional cerebral metabolic alterations in dementia of the Alzheimer type. Positron emission tomography with [^{18}F]-fluorodeoxyglucose. J Comp Assist Tomogr 7:590–598

Friedland RP, Prusiner SB, Jagust WJ, Budinger TF, Davis RL (1984) Bitemporal hypometabolism in Creutzfeldt-Jakob disease measured by positron emission tomography with ^{18}F-fluorodeoxyglucose. J Comp Asst Tomogr 8:978–981

Grady CL, Haxby JV, Horwitz C, Berg G, Rapoport SI (1987) Neuropsychological and cerebral metabolic function in early vs late onset dementia of the Alzheimer type. Neuropsychologia 5:807–816

Gustafson L (1987) Frontal lobe degeneration of non-Alzheimer type II – clinical picture and differential diagnosis. Arch Gerontol Geriatr 6:209–223

Haxby JV, Duara R, Grady CL, Cutler NR, Rapoport SI (1985) Relations between neuropsychological and cerebral metabolic asymmetries in early Alzheimer's disease. J Cereb Blood Flow Metab 5:193–200

Heyman A, Wilkinson WE, Stafford JA, Helms MJ, Sigmon AH, Weinberg T (1984) Alzheimer's disease: a study of epidemiological aspects. Ann Neurol 15:335–341

Jagust WJ, Friedland RP, Budinger TF, Koss E, Ober B (1988) Longitudinal studies of regional cerebral metabolism in Alzheimer's disease. Neurology 38:909–912

Kamo H, McGeer PL, Harrop R, McGeer EG, Calne DB, Martin LRW, Pate BD (1987) Positron emission tomography and histopathology in Pick's disease. Neurology 37:439–445

Kirshner HS, Webb WG, Kelly MP, Wells CE (1984) Language disturbance as an initial symptom of cortical degeneration and dementia. Arch Neurol 41:491–496

Kirshner HS, Tarridag O, Thurman L, Whetsell WO (1987) Progressive aphasia without dementia: two cases with focal spongiform degeneration. Ann Neurol 22:527–532

Leenders KL, Palmer AJ, Quinn N, et al. (1986) Brain dopamine metabolism in patients with Parkinson's disease studied with positron emission tomography. J Neurol Neurosurg Psychiatr 49:853–860

Mayeux R, Stern Y, Spanton S (1985) Heterogeneity in dementia of the Alzheimer type. Neurology 35:453–461

McKenna P, Warrington EK (1983) Graded naming test. NFER-Nelson Publishing Co Ltd, Windsor Berks

McKhann G, Drachman D, Folstein M, Katzman R, Price D, Stadlan EM (1984) Clinical diagnosis of Alzheimer's disease: report of the NINCDS-ARDA work groups under the auspices of Department of Health and Human Services task force on Alzheimer's disease. Neurology 34:939–944

Mesulam MM (1982) Slowly progressive aphasia without generalised dementia. Ann Neurol II:592–598

Molsa PK, Marttila RJ, Rinne UK (1984) Extrapyramidal signs in Alzheimer's disease. Neurology 34:1114–1116

Morris JC, Drazner M, Fulling K, Grant EA, Goldring J (1989) Clinical and pathological aspects of Parkinsonism in Alzheimer's disease. A role for extranigral factors? Arch Neurol 46:651–657

Neary D, Snowden JS, Northern B, Goulding P (1988) Dementia of frontal lobe type. J Neurol Neurosurg Psychiatr 51:353–361

Patlak CS, Blasberg RG (1985) Graphical evaluation of blood-to-brain transfer constants from multiple-time uptake data. Generalisations. J Cereb Blood Flow Metab 5:584–590

Poeck K, Luzzati C (1988) Slowly progressive aphasia in three patients: the problem of accompanying neuropsychological deficit. Brain III:151–168

Polinsky RJ, Noble H, Di Chiro G, Nee LE, Feldman RG, Brown RT (1987) Dominantly inherited Alzheimer's disease: cerebral glucose metabolism. J Neurol Neurosurg Psychiatr 50:752–757

Rossor MN, Iversen LL, Reynolds GP, Mountjoy CQ, Roth M (1984) Neurochemical characteristics of early and late onset types of Alzheimer's disease. Br Med J 288:961–964

Seltzer B, Sherwin I (1983) A comparison of clinical features in early- and late-onset primary degenerative dementia. Arch Neurol 40:143–146

Small GW, Kuhl DE, Riege WH, Fujikawa DG, Ashford JW, Metter EJ, Mazziotta JC (1989) Cerebral glucose metabolic patterns in Alzheimer's disease. Effect of gender and age at dementia onset. Arch Ger Psychiat 46:527–532

Sorbi S, Bracco L, Piacentini S, Moradi A, Amaducci L (1984) Chemical lateralisation in human temporal cortex. Monog Neural Sci II:157–162

Tyrrell P, Rossor M (1988) The association of gegenhalten in the upper limbs with dyspraxia. J Neurol Neurosurg Psychiatr 51:995–997

Tyrrell PJ, Rossor MN (1989) Extrapyramidal signs in dementia of the Alzheimer type. Lancet 2:920

Tyrrell PJ, Warrington EK, Frackowiak RSJ, Rossor MN (1989a) Heterogeneity in progressive dysphasia due to focal cortical atrophy: a clinical and PET study. Brain, in press

Tyrrell PJ, Rossor MN, Frackowiak RSJ (1989b) Oxygen metabolism in degenerative dementia, in press

Warrington EK, McCarthy RA (1988) Fractionation of retrograde amnesia. Brain and Cognition 7:184–200

Cortical Functional Impairment in Dementia of the Alzheimer Type: Studies with Positron Emission Tomography

J. C. Baron

The study of cortical function by positron emission tomography can be approached by measuring local energy metabolism, blood flow, protein synthesis rates and tissue pH (Baron 1986a). In addition, several functional parameters related to neurotransmission are already available (e.g., studies of receptor function, dopamine reuptake sites [^{18}F]fluoro-L-DOPA presynaptic accumulation), while others are still under investigation (e.g., choline uptake, activity of specific enzymes). However, studies in dementia of the Alzheimer type (DAT) have until now mainly concentrated on energy metabolism, because metabolic rates of glucose or oxygen provide a reliable index of local synaptic activity. These studies have opened up new concepts in the pathophysiology of cortical dysfunction in DAT and, at the same time, have allowed a better differentiation in vivo among the various types of senile dementia.

General Observations

In patients meeting the NINCDS criteria for probable dementia of the Alzheimer type (DAT) and moderate-to-severe dementia, there is an overall reduction in cortical energy metabolism (De Leon et al. 1983; Duara et al. 1986; Frackowiak et al. 1981; McGeer et al. 1986a). Regionally, there is a consistent predominance of this metabolic depression over the parieto-occipital associative cortex (Cutler et al. 1985a, b; Duara et al. 1986; Foster et al. 1983, 1984; Frackowiak et al. 1981; Friedland et al. 1983, 1985; Kuhl et al. 1983; McGeer et al. 1986b). The prefrontal cortex is relatively less affected, but the premotor cortex appears markedly involved (Haxby et al. 1988). The primary sensory motor and visual cortices are essentially spared metabolically. The medial temporal areas have been difficult to study with positron emission tomography (PET) due to limited spatial resolution, but recent studies using high-resolution devices have reported significant metabolic reductions in these cortical areas, to a lesser extent, however, than corresponding lateral temporal areas (Foster et al. 1988). Finally, the metabolic rates of the basal ganglia, thalamus and cerebellum are essentially normal except in advanced stages of DAT.

In autopsy-proven cases of Alzheimer's disease (AD), the same pattern of regional metabolic depression was present during life (McGeer et al. 1986b; Haxby et al. 1988). In nine of ten such subjects studied by PET 9–70 months prior to death, Foster et al. (1989) reported an individually significant posterior temporoparietal hypometabolic pattern; in one case, however, the prefrontal cortex was the most hypometabolic cortical area.

These major metabolic changes in DAT have been characterized using age-matched subjects as controls, indicating that a conspicuous distinction exists between DAT and normal aging as revealed by metabolic PET studies. "Supernormal" healthy aging is not associated with any change in brain glucose metabolic rate, while in "normal" aging there is a mild diffuse reduction in cortical metabolism which appears to slightly predominate in the frontal lobe (Kuhl et al. 1982; Baron 1988 a).

Statistically significant cortical metabolic *asymmetries* are frequently observed in probable DAT, as compared to normal subjects in whom the metabolic values are quite symmetrical in baseline conditions (Foster et al. 1983, 1984; Friedland et al. 1985; Grady et al. 1986). These metabolic asymmetries in probable DAT are especially prominent over the posterior associative cortical areas as well as in the prefrontal cortex. In ten autopsy-proven cases, Foster et al. (1989) reported significant cortical metabolic asymmetries in four cases, with the right hemisphere being more affected in three and the left in one. In 31 patients with probable DAT, Loewenstein et al. (1989) reported a significantly greater proportion of left-sided cortical glucose hypometabolism than in controls, particularly in the frontal lobe; a similar left predominance of effects was seen in multi-infarct dementia.

The left-right asymmetries in cortical energy metabolism in DAT have been observed to linearly correlate in a positive way to thalamic, and in a negative way to cerebellar, left-right metabolic ratios (Akiyama et al. 1989). These metabolic changes in the ipsilateral thalamus and contralateral cerebellum that occur in proportion to the depression of cortical metabolism have been interpreted as remote (trans-synaptic) metabolic effects, according to the concept of diaschisis (Baron 1987).

Time Course of Effects

Transversal studies of probable DAT have shown that the metabolic impairment in the cortex tends to both spread and worsen as a function of dementia severity (Cutler et al. 1985a; Duara et al. 1986; Haxby et al. 1987, 1988; Jagust et al. 1988). In mildly demented cases, the cortical hypometabolism is significant only over the superior parietal cortex, while it is also present over the lateral temporal, premotor and anterior occipital cortex in moderately demented cases, and over the prefontal cortex in severely demented cases (Cutler et al. 1985a; Duara et al. 1986; Haxby et al. 1988). Of interest has been the study of early cases where the functional impairment was so mild as to allow only a diagnosis of possible DAT. In these patients, in whom the deficit was mainly confined to memory, a significant parietal cortex hypometabolism was already present (Haxby et al. 1986, 1988; Kuhl et al. 1987) and was found to aggravate as DAT was longitudinally confirmed, suggesting that parietal hypometabolism represents an early marker of the disease (Haxby et al. 1987). In moderately demented DAT cases, longitudinal follow-up has demonstrated both an accentuation of the posterior metabolic depression and a trend for reduction of initially present cortical metabolic asymmetries that were correlated to the decline in intellectual functions (Cutler et al. 1985b; Grady et al. 1986; Haxby et al. 1987; Jagust et al. 1988).

The posterior predominance of cortical hypometabolism typical of early cases tends to disappear in moderately demented patients as premotor-prefrontal metabolism deteriorates (Haxby et al. 1988). In advanced DAT cases, a pattern of predominantly frontal hypometabolism has been reported (Benson et al. 1983; Frackowiak et al. 1981; Metter et al. 1985). Except in the case of one such patient, who was proven by postmortem study to have AD (Foster et al. 1989), neuropathological diagnosis has been lacking.

Clinical Subtypes

Only two studies have compared presenile to senile DAT. Koss et al. (1985) reported a predominantly left parietal hypometabolism in presenile DAT, whereas it predominated over the right side in senile cases. Grady et al. (1987), who adequately matched their patients for both duration and severity of dementia, observed that the parietal posterior hypometabolic pattern typical of DAT was significantly more apparent in presenile than in senile cases.

The brain metabolic pattern typical of sporadic cases of probable DAT has been reproduced in studies of familial AD, indicating a lack of differential metabolic impairment between these two clinical categories (Polinsky et al. 1987; Hoffmann et al. 1989). In one patient with Down's syndrome and autopsy-proven AD, Schapiro et al. (1988) similarly reported a pattern of brain hypometabolism typical of DAT.

Correlations with Neuropsychological Impairment

This topic is the subject of a specific chapter in this volume by Haxby et al. The data can be summarized in the following way. Whether by selecting DAT patients with clearly lateralized neuropsychological impairment, or by comparing in nonselected DAT cases the left-right cortical metabolic asymmetries to the "pattern" of neuropsychological impairment (assessed by designing left-right indexes such as verbal-versus-visuospatial neuropsychological scores), investigators have consistently reported highly significant correlations between metabolic changes in the cortex and cognitive impairment. Hence, the posterior associative cortex hypometabolism is associated with a predominance of the neuropsychological impairment in the verbal tasks when it affects, the left (dominant) hemisphere more, and in the visuospatial tasks when it affects the right hemisphere more (Foster et al. 1983, 1986; Grady et al. 1986; Haxby et al. 1985, 1986). In patients with predominant memory impairment, the cortical metabolic impairment is essentially symmetrical (Foster et al. 1983). In pure amnesia cases, however, an asymmetric posterior parietal hypometabolism has been reported, which lacked any detectable neocortical neuropsychological counterpart; at follow-up, however, these cases proved to develop DAT with now correspondingly lateralized neuropsychologic deficit, indicating that the metabolic impairment actually preceded the related clinical manifestation (Haxby et al. 1986, 1987). Initial accounts on medial temporal cortex metabolism measured by high-resolution PET in DAT have appeared (Foster et al. 1988); they indicate less impairment than in the lateral temporal cortex, but correlations with memory task performance are still lacking. Metabolic asymmetries in the prefontal cortex appear to correlate with a neuropsychological left-right index similar to those in the parietal cortex (Haxby et al. 1986). However, anteroposterior metabolic ratios, such as parietal/premotor or parietal/prefrontal, have been found to correlate significantly with verbal-visual over attention-fluency ratio indexes (Haxby et al. 1988). Obviously, a lot of work remains to be done in this area with respect to the resting pattern of brain metabolism, while the more difficult study of the metabolic responses to cognitive tasks in DAT has only recently been tackled (Miller et al. 1987).

Clinical Diagnostic Implications

The consistency in the brain metabolic pattern seen in DAT suggests PET (or SPECT) imaging of cerebral blood flow, a parameter coupled to energy metabolism in DAT (Frackowiak et al. 1981; Duara et al. 1989), could be used to help diagnose DAT in the clinic. However, the patients investigated so far by PET have been part of research protocols, which include only that small proportion of demented patients who meet the research criteria for DAT. Ideally, sensitivity and specificity studies of metabolic brain imaging for the diagnosis of DAT should enroll, in separate trials, early, mid-stage, and end-stage demented patients presenting consecutively to the clinic and should theoretically include final neuropathologic diagnostic classifications such as AD, MID, mixed AD-MID, and Pick's disease. In such trials, it is the *individual* diagnostic value of PET that will have to be determined. These types of trials will also help retrospectively establish "atypical" patterns of brain metabolism in autopsy-confirmed AD in a search for disease subtypes or variants (Foster et al. 1989). Finally, specific prospective studies comparing "pseudo-dementia" due to depression to probable DAT are warranted (Kuhl et al. 1983). To date, however, the typical pattern of predominantly posterior parietal hypometabolism has only been reported in demented patients with Parkinson's disease (Kuhl et al. 1985), in whom an association with authentic AD is likely. Highly focal hypometabolism in right parietal and left temporal cortex has been reported in still unclassified patients with left arm impairment and constructive apraxia (Bolgert et al. 1989) or isolated progressive aphasia (Chawluk et al. 1986a; Tyrrell et al. 1989), respectively.

Pathophysiologic Considerations

Since the metabolic pattern of individual DAT patients is remarkably repro-
ducible over time (Grady et al. 1986; Jagust et al. 1988), the inference is that it
must reflect a permanent impairment of the neuronal circuits involved, which
could reflect either neuronal death per se, or a neuronal dysfunction (e.g., as a
result of "deactivation" or disconnection), or both. Three major facts favor the
neuronal loss hypothesis: (1) cortical atrophy, which is significantly increased in
DAT relative to aged controls (Creasy et al., this volume) if taken into account in
the PET procedure, would account for part of the hypometabolic pattern seen
(Chawluk et al. 1986b; Herscovitch et al. 1986); (2) the distribution of the hypometabolic pattern typical of early DAT is roughly superimposable on that
noted postmortem for neurofibrillary tangles (Brun and Englund 1986); and (3)
this pattern is also similar to that of the decrease in cortical somatostatin seen
postmortem (Tamminga et al. 1987; Procter et al. 1988). Hence, the PET procedure would provide in vivo a mapping of the neuronal lesions in the cortex that
could be used as a useful index in the long-term assessment of putative therapy.

However, the above facts should be qualified. For example, detailed PET-neu-
ropathology confrontations have been reported for only two cases (McGeer et al.
1986b; Schapiro et al. 1988), and the posterior association cortex is also the site
of maximum decreases in the enzyme choline acetyltransferase (ChAT) (Procter
et al. 1988), which is a marker of basalocortical cholinergic terminals. Also, the
frequent metabolic involvement of the premotor and prefrontal cortex in DAT
seems out of proportion to the cortical neuropathology usually observed there.
Hence, a contribution of neuronal deactivation disconnection in the cortical
metabolic impairment observed by PET should be considered seriously. Such a
hypothesis would imply that the dysfunctional cortical neurons would still re-
spond to treatment aimed at restoring transmission within, or enhancing adaptive
mechanisms of, deafferented fields (by means of, e.g., transmitter precursors,
grafting, growth factors). Mechanisms for these effects would entail dysfunction
of (1) intrinsic or corticocortical circuits; (2) corticosubcorticocortical loops; and
(3) subcorticocortical projection systems (Fig. 1). Evidence for the last two mechanisms is available. Hence, it has been clearly shown that in patients with DAT
the cortical metabolic asymmetries are significantly correlated to similar basal-
ganglia-thalamus, and to reverse cerebellar asymmetries, according to the concept of (slowly evolving) diaschisis (Akiyama et al. 1989). A transneuronally
mediated effect through the corticostriatopallidothalamocortical loop could then
secondarily aggravate the cortical dysfunction. Hypometabolism of the cerebral
cortex, associated to behavioral impairment, has been clearly demonstrated in
lesions of the striatum, the pallidum and the thalamus (Metter et al. 1986;
Laplane et al. 1989; Baron et al. 1986b; Levasseur et al. 1989). In addition, the
usually minor direct neuronal lesions in these latter structures may be prominent
in subtypes of AD. With respect to the subcorticocortical projecting systems,
lesions of the nucleus basalis of Meynert (NbM), the raphé system and the locus
coeruleus (LC) are essentially constant in AD. The role of the cholinergic input
in the functional activity of the cerebral cortex is well known from electrophysiological, pharmacological and behavioral studies. Cholinergic enhancers (e.g.,

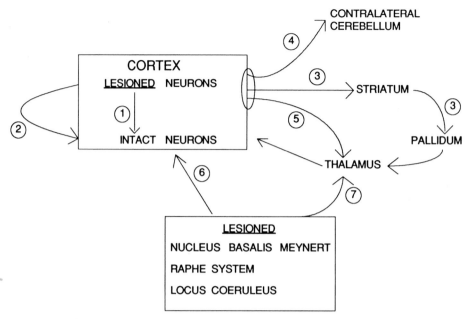

Fig. 1. Potentially disconnected circuits in AD leading to deafferentiation of cortical neurons: *1*, intrinsic cortical neurons; *2*, corticocortical systems; *3*, corticostriatopallidothalamocortical loop; *4*, corticopontocerebellar pathway; *5*, corticothalamic fibers; *6*, subcorticocortical ascending systems; *7*, thalamic afferents from cholinergic 5-HT and norepinephrine system

muscarinic agonists, acetylcholinesterase blockers) increase, and muscarinic antagonists decrease, cortical glucose utilization in animals (Baron 1988 b). Unilateral lesions of the NbM or its equivalent in rats and baboons induce a marked ipsilateral depression of cortical glucose use (London et al. 1984; Orzi et al. 1986; Kiyosawa et al. 1987, 1989). These facts constitute strong evidence for a role of the NbM lesions in the cortical hypometabolism of DAT and put a case in favor of cholinergic enhancers in DAT, while additional effects could proceed through the basalothalamic cholinergic pathway. A disturbing factor in this hypothesis comes from the consistent observation, made both in rats and in baboons, of an effective metabolic recovery despite persisting deficit in cortical ChAT activity (Kiyosawa et al. 1989). It remains possible, however, that such an efficient process of adaptation to cholinergic deafferentation – be it presynaptic, postsynaptic or even transneuronal – could be absent in bilaterally lesioned, aged animals or in combined NbM-raphe-LC lesioned animals, all situations that would more closely mimic the human disease.

Finally, periventricular white matter lesions of an apparently vascular nature have been reported postmortem in AD (Englund et al. 1988). These lesions could further disconnect the overlying cortical regions from afferents of the kinds discussed above and hence result in accentuated hypometabolism (Baron 1990). Although no specific study of this issue has appeared yet, the available PET literature on leuko-araïosis (Delpla et al. 1989) and experimental corpus callosum section in baboons (Yamaguchi et al. 1989) indicates that this is a hypothesis worthy of consideration.

References

Akiyama H, Harrop R, McGeer PL, Reppart R, McGeer EG (1989) Crossed cerebellar and uncrossed basal ganglia and thalamic diaschisis in Alzheimer's disease. Neurology 39:451–548

Baron JC (1986a) New perspectives in functional imaging of the aging brain. In: Courtois Y, Faucheux B, Forette B, Knook DL, Treton JA (eds) Modern trends in aging research. Libbey, Paris, 147:459–467

Baron JC, d'Antona R, Pantano P, Serdaru M, Samson Y, Bousser MG (1986b) Effects of thalamic stroke on energy metabolism in the cerebral cortex. Brain 109:1234–1259

Baron JC (1987) Remote metabolic effects of stroke. In: Wade J, Knezevic S, Maximilian VA, Mubrin Z, Prokovnik I (eds) Impact of functional imaging in neurology and psychiatry. London, John Libbey, 91–100

Baron JC (1988a) Etude in vivo du métabolisme cérébral énergétique au cours du vieillissement cérébral normal. In: "Le vieillissement cérébral normal et pathologique", Fondation Nationale de Gérontologie, pp 190–199

Baron JC (1988b) Système cholinergique et métabolisme énergétique cérébral. Cir Metabol Cerveau 5:183–189

Baron JC (1990) Substance blanche, métabolisme cérébral et vieillissement. In: Bes A, Geraud G (eds) Circulation cérébrale et vieillissement. Springer, Berlin Heidelberg New York, in press

Benson DF, Kuhl DE, Hawkins RA, Phelps ME, Cumming JL, Tsai SY (1983) The fluorodeoxyglucose ^{18}F scan in Alzheimer's disease and multi-infarct dementia. Arch Neurol 40:711–714

Bolgert F, Leger JM, Levasseur M, Benoit N, Samson Y, Baron JC, Signoret JL (1989) Slowly progressive right parietal lobe: clinical MRI, and PET scan findings in three cases. Neurology 39 (suppl 1):181

Brun A, Englund E (1986) Brain changes in dementia of Alzheimer's type relevant to new imaging methods. Prog Neuro-psychopharmacol Biol Psychiat 10:297–308

Chawluk JB, Mesulam MM, Hartig H, et al. (1986b) Slowly progressive aphasia without generalized dementia: studies with positron emission tomography. Ann Neurol 19:68–74

Chawluk JB, Alavi A, Dann E, et al. (1986a) Positron emission tomography in aging and dementia: effect of cerebral atrophy. J Nucl Med 28:431–437

Cutler NR, Haxby JB, Duara R, et al. (1985a) Clinical history, brain metabolism and neuropsychological function in Alzheimer's disease. Ann Neurol 18:298–309

Cutler NR, Haxby JB, Duara R, et al. (1985b) Brain metabolism as measured by positron emission tomography. Neurology 35:1556–1561

DeLeon MF, Ferris SH, George AE, Reisberg B, Christman DR, Krischeff SS, Wolf AP (1983) Computed tomography and positron emission transaxial tomography evaluations of normal aging and Alzheimer's disease. J Cereb Blood Flow Metabol 3:391–394

Delpla P, Meyer E, Zatone R, et al. (1989) Metabolic and neuropsychological correlates of periventricular lucencies. J Cereb Blood Flow Metabol 9 (suppl 1):S569

Duara R, Grady C, Haxby J, Sundaram M, Cutler NR, Heston L, Moore A, Schilegeter N, Larson S, Rapoport SI (1986) Positron emission tomography in Alzheimer's disease. Neurology 36:879–887

Duara R, Barker W, Pascal S, Chang JY, Apicella A, Ginsberg M (1989) The coupling of cerebral blood flow and metabolism in Alzheimer's disease and multi-infarct dementia. J Cereb Blood Flow Metabol (suppl) 9:S538

Englund E, Brun A, Alling C (1988) White matter changes in dementia of Alzheimer's type. Brain 11:1425–1439

Foster NL, Chase TN, Fedio P, Patronas NJ, Brooks RA, Di Chiro G (1983) Alzheimer's disease: local cortical changes shown by positron emission tomography. Neurology 33:961–965

Foster NL, Chase TN, Mansi L, Brooks R, Fedio P, Patronas NJ, Di Chiro G (1984) Cortical abnormalities in Alzheimer's disease. Ann Neurol 16:649–654

Foster NL, Chase TN, Patronas NJ, Gillespie MM, Fedio P (1986) Cerebral mapping of apraxia in Alzheimer's disease by positron emission tomography. Ann Neurol 19:139–143

Foster NL, Hansen MS, Siegel GJ, Kuhl DE (1988) Mesial and lateral temporal glucose metabolism in aging and Alzheimer's disease studied by PET. Neurology 38 (suppl. 1):133

Foster NL, Mann U, Mohr E, Sunderland T, Katz D, Chase TN (1989) Focal cerebral glucose hypometabolism in definite Alzheimer's disease. Ann Neurol 26:132–133

Frackowiak RSJ, Pozzilli C, Legg NJ, du Boulay GH, Marshall J, Lenzi GL, Jones T (1981) Regional cerebral oxygen supply and utilization in dementia: a clinical and physiological study with oxygen-15 and positron tomography. Brain 104:753–778

Friedland RP, Budinger TF, Ganz E, Yano Y, Mathis CA, Koss B, Ober BA, Huesman RH (1983) Regional cerebral metabolic alterations in dementia of Alzheimer type: positron emission tomography with 18F-fluorodeoxyglucose. J Computer Assist Tomography 7:590–598

Friedland RP, Budinger TF, Koss E, Ober BA (1985) Alzheimer's disease: anterior-posterior and lateral hemispheric alteration in cortical glucose utilization. Neurosci Lett 53:235–240

Grady CL, Haxby JV, Horwitz B, Berg G, Rapoport SI (1987) Neuropsychological and cerebral metabolic function in early vs late onset dementia of the Alzheimer type. Neuropsychologia 25:807–816

Grady CL, Haxby JV, Schlageter NL, Berg G, Rapoport SI (1986) Stability of metabolic and neuropsychological asymmetries in dementia of the Alzheimer's type. Neurology 36:1390–1392

Haxby JV, Duara R, Graby CL, Cutler NR, Rapoport SI (1985) Relations between neuropsychological and cerebral metabolic asymmetries in early Alzheimer's disease. J Cereb Blood Flow Metabol 5:193–200

Haxby JV, Grady CL, Duara R, Schlageter N, Berg G, Rapoport SI (1986) Neocortical metabolic abnormalities precede non memory cognitive defects in early Alzheimer's type dementia. Arch Neurol 43:882–885

Haxby JV, Grady CL, Friedland RP, Rapoport SI (1987) Neocortical metabolic abnormalities precede nonmemory cognitive impairments in early dementia of the Alzheimer type: longitudinal confirmation. J Neurol Trans 24 (suppl):49–53

Haxby JV, Grady CL, Koss E, Horwitz B, Schapiro M, Friedland RP, Rapoport SI (1988) Heterogeneous anterior-posterior metabolic patterns in dementia of the Alzheimer type. Neurology 38:1853–1863

Herscovitch F, Auchus AP, Gado M, Chi D, Raichle ME (1986) Correction of positron emission tomography data for cerebral atrophy. J Cereb Blood Flow Metabol 6:120–124

Hoffman JM, Guze BH, Baxter L, Hawk TC, Frijikawa DJ, Dorsey D, Maltese A, Small G, Mazziotta JC, Kuhl DE (1989) Familial and sporadic Alzheimer's disease: an FDG-PET study. J Cereb Blood Flow Metabol 9 (suppl):S547

Jagust WJ, Friedland RP, Budinger TF, Koss E, Ober B (1988) Longitudinal studies of regional cerebral metabolism in Alzheimer's disease. Neurology 38:909–912

Kiyosawa M, Pappata S, Duverger D, et al. (1987) Cortical hypometabolism and its recovery following nucleus basalis lesions in baboons: a PET study. J Cereb Blood Flow Metabol 7:812–817

Kiyosawa M, Baron JC, Hamel E, et al. (1989) Time course of effects of unilateral lesions of the nucleus basalis of Meynert on glucose utilization of the cerebral cortex: positron tomography in baboons. Brain 112:435–455

Koss E, Friedland RP, Ober BA, Jagust WJ (1985) Differences in lateral hemispheric asymmetries of glucose utilization between early and late-onset Alzheimer's type dementia. Am J Psychiat 142:638–640

Kuhl DE, Metter EJ, Riege WH, Hawkins RA, Mazziotta JC, Phelps ME, Kling AS (1983) Local cerebral glucose utilization in elderly patients with depression, multiple infarct dementia and Alzheimer's disease. J Cereb Blood Flow Metabol 3 (suppl 1):494–495

Kuhl DE, Metter EJ, Riege WH, Phelps ME (1982) Effects of human aging on patterns of local cerebral glucose utilization determined by the [18F] Fluorodeoxyglucose method. J Cereb Blood Flow Metabol 2:163–171

Kuhl DE, Metter EJ, Benson F, Wesson-Ashford J, Riege WH, Fujikawa DG, Markham CH, et al. (1985) Similarities of cerebral glucose metabolism in Alzheimer's disease and Parkinsonian dementia. J Cereb Blood Flow Metabol 5 (suppl 1):169–170

Kuhl DE, Small GW, Riege WH, et al. (1987) Cerebral metabolic patterns before the diagnosis of probable Alzheimer's disease. J Cereb Blood Flow Metabol 7 (suppl 1):406

Laplane D, Levasseur M, Pillon B, Dubois B, Baulac M, Mazoyer B, Tran Dinh S, Sette G, Danze F, Baron JC (1989) Obsessive-compulsive and other behavioral changes with bilateral basal ganglia lesions: a neuropsychological magnetic resonance imaging and positron emission tomography study. Brain 112:699–725

Levasseur M, Mazoyer B, Sette G, Legault-Demare F, Pappata S, Maugière F, Benoit N, Tran-Dinh S, Baron JC (1989) Bilateral paramedian thalamic infarction: a PET study of cortical oxygen consumption. J Cereb Blood Flow Metab 9 (suppl):738

Loewenstein DA, Barker WA, Chang JY, Apicella A, Yoshii F, Kothari P, Levin B, Duara R (1989) Predominant left hemisphere metabolic dysfunction in dementia. Arch Neurol 46:146–152

London ED, McKinney M, Dam M, Ellis A, Coyle TJ (1984) Decreased cortical glucose utilization after ibotenate lesions of the rat ventromedial globus pallidus. J Cereb Blood Flow Metabol 4:381–390

McGeer PL, Kamo H, Harrop R, Li DKB, Tuokko H, McGeer EG, Adam MJ, Amman W (1986a) Positron emission tomography in patients with clinically diagnosed Alzheimer's disease. Can Med Assoc J 134:597–607

McGeer PL, Kamo H, Harrop R, McGeer EG, Martin WRW, Pate DB, Li DKB (1986b) Comparison of PET, MRI and CT with pathology in a proven case of Alzheimer's disease. Neurology 36:1569–1574

Metter EJ, Riege WH, Benson DF, Phelps ME, Kuhl DE (1985) Variability of regional cerebral glucose metabolism in Alzheimer's disease patients as compared to controls. J Cereb Metabol 5 (suppl 1):127–128

Metter EJ, Jackson C, Kempler D, et al. (1986) Left hemisphere intracerebral hemorrhages studied by F-18-Fluorodeoxyglucose PET. Neurology 36:1155–1162

Miller JD, Deleon MJ, Ferris SH, et al. (1987) Abnormal temporal lobe response in Alzheimer's disease during cognitive processing as measured by 14C-2-Deoxyglucose and PET. J Cereb Blood Flow Metabol 7:248–251

Orzi F, Diana G, Palombo E, Lenzi GL, Bracco L, Fieschi C (1986) Effects of unilateral lesion of the nucleus basalis on local cerebral glucose utilization in rat. In: Vezzadin P, et al. (eds) Neuroendocrine system and aging. Roma, Eurage Publisher, pp 259–264

Polinsky RJ, Noble H, Di Chiro G, Nee LE, Feldman RG, Brown RT (1987) Dominantly inherited Alzheimer's disease: cerebral glucose metabolism. J Neurol Neurosurg Psychiat 50:752–757

Procter AW, Lowe SL, Palmer AM et al. (1988) Topographical distribution of neurochemical changes in Alzheimer's disease. J Neurol Sci 84:125–140

Schapiro MB, Ball MJ, Grady CL, Haxby JV, Kaye JA, Rapoport SI (1988) Dementia in Down's syndrome. Neurology 38:938–942

Tamminga CA, Foster NL, Fedio P, Bird E, Chase TN (1987) Alzheimer's disease: low cerebral somatostatin levels correlate with impaired cognitive function and cortical metabolism. Neurology 37:161–165

Tyrrell PJ, Perani D, Warrington EK, Frackowiak RSJ, Rossor MN (1989) Slowly progressive aphasia with and without dementia: metabolic studies with PET. J Cereb Blood Flow Metabol 9 (suppl):S514

Yamaguchi T, Kunimoto M, Pappata S, et al. (1989) Effects of anterior corpus callosum section on cortical glucose utilization in baboons: a sequential positron emission tomography study. Brain, in press

Brain Imaging with SPECT in Alzheimer's Disease

G. Waldemar, O. B. Paulson and N. A. Lassen

Summary

Alzheimer's disease is associated with reductions of regional cerebral blood flow and metabolism. Since the development of the ^{133}Xe inhalation technique for tomographic measurements of regional cerebral blood flow, single photon emission computer tomography (SPECT) of the brain has played an important role in the study of dementia disorders. Recently, hexamethyl-propylene-amine-oxime (*d,l*-HMPAO) for labeling with ^{99m}Tc was developed as a tracer for regional blood flow distribution studies by SPECT.

In an angoing study of [^{99m}Tc]HMPAO SPECT in dementia and normal aging, 18 patients fulfilled the clinical criteria for "probable Alzheimer's disease." In 17 patients the regional cerebral blood flow pattern was rated as abnormal by visual inspection. In eight patients regional cerebral blood flow was reduced primarily in posterior temporoparietal regions. In four patients regional cerebral blood flow was reduced primarily in the frontal lobe, although often with some temporal lobe involvement, and in five patients frontal and posterior areas were equally affected. These changes were not associated with any focal parenchymal changes in the X-ray computer tomography (CT) scans. The diverse localizations of regional cerebral blood flow reductions were in good agreement with the clinical symptoms, and may reflect different subgroups or stages of Alzheimer's disease.

Brain imaging with SPECT provides functional information correlative to neuropsychological data and may be helpful in evaluating treatment effects and prognosis. However, only studies with repeated evaluations of patients until neuropathological confirmation of the diagnosis will reveal the exact diagnostic and prognostic value of SPECT in Alzheimer's disease.

Introduction

Alzheimer's disease is associated with reductions of regional cerebral blood flow and metabolism. Tomographic measurements of regional cerebral blood flow with single photon emission computer tomography (SPECT) were first made possible by the ^{133}Xe inhalation technique (Celsis et al. 1981; Stokely et al. 1980).

This method facilitates repetitive quantitative studies and, hence, vasoactive stress tests, which in some patients may contribute important information for the differential diagnosis of dementia. However, the technique requires special SPECT equipment and is associated with some drawbacks, such as artifacts due to the high concentration of ^{133}Xe in the nasal airways and a low resolution, which to some extent limit its use in the regional mapping of dementia disorders. New ^{99m}Tc-labeled tracers, which are trapped in the brain as a function of the blood flow, have been designed for SPECT. Hexamethyl-propylene-amine-oxime (d,l-HMPAO) for labeling with ^{99m}Tc is one such new radiopharmaceutical introduced as a tracer for cerebral blood flow (Neirinckx et al. 1987; Andersen et al. 1988). In the brain it is rapidly converted to a hydrophilic form which is retained for several hours. The steady-state distribution in the brain is almost proportional to regional cerebral blood flow. Therefore, imaging of tracer uptake in the brain may be performed using a conventional rotating gamma camera, and with a dedicated SPECT camera a very high resolution is attained. Thus, although no follow-up studies have been performed, [^{99m}Tc]HMPAO SPECT could play a widespread and important role in the routine differential diagnosis of dementia, and in the subgrouping and prognostic rating of patients with Alzheimer's disease.

This paper discusses the use of SPECT as a functional neuroimaging technique in relation to dementia of the Alzheimer type. A preliminary report on patterns of regional cerebral blood flow abnormalities in a group of 18 patients with probable Alzheimer's disease is included.

Patients

Eighteen patients with dementia of the Alzheimer type, according to the NINCDS-ADRDA criteria (McKhann et al. 1984) for "probable Alzheimer's disease," were studied. The median age was 70 years (range, 58–83 years), and the median duration of disease was 3 years (range, 0.5–10 years). All patients underwent an extensive study program – including at least one interview of the patient and relatives, neurological examination, neuropsychological tests, laboratory tests, and a computer tomography (CT) scan – to exclude other possible causes of dementia. The CT scans were all normal, except for atrophy. The severity of dementia was graded by the Mini-Mental-State (Folstein et al. 1975), which has a maximum score of 30. The median Mini-Mental-State score was 16 (range, 3–27). Informed consent to participate in the study, which was approved by the local ethical committee, was obtained from the patient and a close relative.

Methods

One vial with unlabeled d,l-HMPAO (Ceretec) was mixed with fresh eluent from a ^{99m}Tc generator in daily use. A 10-ml bolus with 1.1 GBq [^{99m}Tc]-d,l-HMPAO

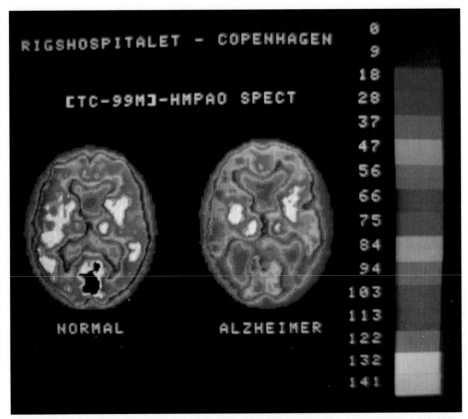

Fig. 1. [^{99m}Tc]HMPAO images 5 cm above the orbitomeatal plane in a 78-year-old healthy volunteer (*left*) and in a 74-year-old patient with Alzheimer's disease (*right*). The *color scale* indicates relative flow units (with the cerebellum as reference region) as explained in the text. The left hemisphere is shown *to the left,* frontal lobe is *at the top.* In the healthy volunteer, note the fairly symmetrical pattern with low subcortical regional cerebral blood flow, due to some central atrophy, surrounded by cortical areas with symmetrically high regional cerebral blood flow. The patient with Alzheimer's disease presented with visual agnosia and memory loss. Regional cerebral blood flow was reduced primarily in posterior temporal (and occipital) regions

was injected intravenously during rest shortly after reconstituting the vial, and approximately 15 min before acquisition of data. Regional cerebral uptake of the tracer was measured by the Tomomatic 64, a rapidly rotating and highly sensitive instrument for SPECT of the brain, described in detail previously (Stokeley et al. 1980). With a high-resolution collimator the resolution in the plane (and the slice thickness) is 10 mm (full width at half maximum, FWHM). Three slices are obtained simultaneously in each study and, by repositioning the patient, a total of nine consecutive slices covering the whole brain may be obtained in parallel to the orbitomeatal plane during three studies. The acquisition time was 20–30 min in each study. Quantification of regional cerebral blood flow relative to mean regional cerebral blood flow in the cerebellum was carried out using the algorithm of Lassen et al. (1988). This algorithm corrects for the contrast-reducing effect of a preferential back-diffusion of tracer from high flow regions over the first 2 min. The validity of this correction procedure, as compared to measurement of regional cerebral blood flow using ^{133}Xe, has been demonstrated previously by Andersen et al. (1988) and also in dementia studies (Waldemar et al. 1988). The regional cerebral blood flow tomograms were blinded and analyzed visually together with tomograms from healthy controls.

Results

In 17 patients the regional cerebral blood flow pattern was sufficiently abnormal to be distinguished from a normal pattern (Fig. 1) by visual inspection alone. In one patient the regional cerebral blood flow image was considered normal for the patient's age. In eight patients regional cerebral blood flow was reduced primarily in posterior temporoparietal regions, and in four patients regional cerebral blood flow was reduced primarily in the frontal lobe, although often with some temporal lobe involvement. In five patients frontal and posterior areas were equally affected. The localizations of regional cerebral blood flow reductions were in good agreement with the clinical symptoms.

Discussion

The in vivo differential diagnosis of the two major causes of dementia – dementia of the Alzheimer type and vascular or multi-infarct dementia – is based on clinical criteria. Although these criteria are still being improved as new validating neuropathological data are obtained, they are still insufficient and overlapping. In research studies, continuing recognition of the assumptions made in the clinical diagnosis of these diseases is important, especially as drugs for possible treatment are becoming available. The methodological difficulties in studies of drug effects in Alzheimer's disease, when based on clinical and psychological evaluations only, are well recognized. Therefore, there is a great need for paraclinical correlates to the reduced cognitive functions in Alzheimer's disease. Such correlates, whether diagnostic for the disease or not, should be easy to measure and sensitive to functional changes in the course of the disease. One important paraclinical correlate to brain function in Alzheimer's disease is regional cerebral blood flow. As seen in the present group of patients, Alzheimer's disease most often is associated with bilateral reductions of regional cerebral blood flow and metabolism in the temporoparietal regions, although often with asymmetric appearance. These changes are not associated with any focal parenchymal changes in the X-ray CT scans.

The application of structural neuroimaging techniques, i.e., conventional X-ray CT and/or magnetic resonance imaging, is necessary in the primary differential diagnosis of the dementia disorders. They may identify small infarcts or white matter disease as the cause of dementia. In the diagnosis of Alzheimer's disease they serve primarily as tools for eliminating other possible (and maybe treatable) causes for the dementia syndrome in each particular patient.

The development of high sensitivity SPECT of inhaled ^{133}Xe (Celsis et al. 1981; Stokely et al. 1980) has increased our understanding of the pathophysiology of cerebrovascular diseases and of global and major regional blood flow changes during normal and abnormal aging of the brain. This method allows for three-dimensional measurement of the uptake and washout of ^{133}Xe from the brain and calculation of regional cerebral blood flow in horizontal slices of the brain. The resolution of this system is 1.5–1.7 cm (FWHM) in the plane with a slice thickness of 2.0 cm. In cases of acute stroke, low-flow areas corresponding to the clinical symptoms are readily seen, and the low flow areas often exceed the areas of complete infarction. The application of the vasoactive stress test, e.g., injection of acetazolamide, provides important additional information on the vascular condition of the tissue in the low flow area (Vorstrup et al. 1986). In dementia this could help identify "vascular" flow defects in areas without complete infarction. In the present group of patients, the result of the acetazolamide stress tests with the ^{133}Xe inhalation technique did not point to a vascular cause for the reduced regional cerebral blood flow (data not presented). In general ^{133}Xe inhalation tomography is easy, repeatable and quantitative, but not compatible with all SPECT instruments.

Over the past few years new radiopharmaceuticals, which are retained in the brain and thus can be used for the study of brain tissue perfusion with static SPECT imaging, have been developed. These compounds are labeled with a suitable isotope and injected intravenously prior to the imaging procedure, which may be performed using a conventional rotating gamma camera, or a dedicated brain SPECT system as the one described above, giving a higher resolution. Isopropyl-iodoamphetamine labeled with ^{123}I was the first compound to be used for static SPECT studies in dementia (Derouesne et al. 1985; Jagust et al. 1987). This method, however, has serious drawbacks owing to early redistribution to low-flow areas, unfavorable dosimetry and high cost.

The compound [^{99m}Tc]-d,l-HMPAO was recently developed as a better "chemical microsphere" for regional blood flow distribution studies by SPECT (Neirinckx et al. 1987). With the brain-dedicated SPECT system, as described above, this compound provides a much higher resolution in the plane (10 mm, FWHM).

The results of the first clinical studies with this tracer in dementia have indicated that a bilaterally reduced uptake in the posterior temporoparietal regions is a striking feature of Alzheimer's disease (Gemmell et al. 1987; Neary et al. 1987; Burns et al. 1989), sufficient to discriminate Alzheimer's disease from multi-infarct dementia (Gemmell et al. 1987). In our experience, however, the results are variable, with occasional flow reductions in the frontal areas as well. This could be due to inclusion of patients fulfilling the Alzheimer's disease criteria, but with possible frontal lobe degeneration of non-Alzheimer type, or it may simply reflect different subgroups of Alzheimer's disease with different primary localizations of the same disease process. In addition, multi-infarct dementia, or vascular dementia, may be associated with several focal abnormalities, often with areas larger than those of the CT changes. In some cases these changes may be symmetric and bilateral as in Alzheimer's disease, leaving the differential diagnosis more difficult.

In conclusion, SPECT of the brain has added a new dimension to our knowledge of the dementia disorders. It provides functional information correlative to neuropsychological data, and may be helpful in evaluating treatment effects and prognosis. However, only studies with repeated evaluations of patients until neuropathological confirmation of the diagnosis will reveal the exact diagnostic and prognostic value of SPECT in Alzheimer's disease.

Acknowledgements. The ongoing study of [^{99m}Tc]HMPAO SPECT in dementia is supported by grants from the Lundbeck Foundation and the Danish Medical Research Council.

References

Andersen AR, Friberg HH, Schmidt JF, Hasselbalch SG (1988) Quantitative measurements of cerebral blood flow using SPECT and [^{99m}Tc]-*d,l*-HM-PAO compared to xenon-133. J Cereb Blood Flow Metab 8:S69–S81

Burns A, Philpot MP, Costa DC, Ell PJ, Levy R (1989) The investigation of Alzheimer's disease with single photon emission tomography. J Neurol Neurosurg Psychiat 52:248–253

Celsis P, Goldman T, Henriksen L, Lassen NA (1981) A method for calculating regional cerebral blood flow from emission computed tomography of inert gas concentrations. J Comp Ass Tomogr 5:641–645

Derouesne C, Rancurel G, Le Poncin Lafitte M, Rapin JR, Lassen NA (1985) Variability of cerebral blood flow defects in Alzheimer's disease on ^{123}Iodo-isopropyl-amphetamine and single photon emission tomography. Lancet i:1282

Folstein MF, Folstein SE, McHugh PR (1975) "Mini-Mental State". A practical method for grading the cognitive state of patients for the clinician. J Psychiat Res 12:189–198

Gemmel HG, Sharp PE, Besson JAO, Crawford JR, Ebmeier KP, Davidson J, Smith FW (1987) Differential diagnosis in dementia using the cerebral blood flow agent ^{99m}Tc HM-PAO: a SPECT study. J Comp Asst Tomogr 11:398–402

Jagust WJ, Budinger TF, Reed BR (1987) The diagnosis of dementia with single photon emisson computed tomography. Arch Neurol 44:258–262

Lassen NA, Andersen AR, Friberg L, Paulson OB (1988) The retention of [^{99m}Tc]-*d,l*-HM-PAO in the human brain after intracarotid bolus injection: a kinetic analysis. J Cereb Blood Flow Metab 8(S1):S13–S22

McKhann G, Drachman D, Folstein M, Katzman R, Price D, Stadlan EM (1984) Clinical diagnosis of Alzheimer's disease: report of the NINCDS-ADRDA work groups under the auspices of Department of Health and Human Services Task Force on Alzheimer's Disease. Neurology 34:939–944

Neary O, Snowdon JS, Shields RA, Burjan AWI, Northen B, MacDermott N, Prescott MC, Testa HJ (1987) Single photon emission tomography using ^{99m}Tc-HM-PAO in the investigation of dementia. J Neurol Neurosurg Psychiat 50:1101–1109

Neirinckx RD, Canning LR, Piper IM, Nowotnik DP, Pickett RD, Holmes RA, Volkert WA, Forster AM, Weisner PS, Marriott JA, Chaplin SB (1987) Technetium-99m *d,l*-HMPAO: a new radiopharmaceutical for SPECT imaging of regional cerebral blood perfusion. J Nucl Med 28:191–202

Stokely EM, Sveinsdottir E, Lassen NA, Rommer P (1980) A single photon dynamic computer assisted tomograph (DCAT) for imaging brain function in multiple cross sections. J Comp Asst Tomogr 4:230–240

Vorstrup S, Brun B, Lassen NA (1986) Evaluation of the cerebral vasodilatory capacity by the acetazolamide test before EC-IC bypass surgery in patients with occlusion of the internal carotid artery. Stroke 17:1291–1298

Waldemar G, Andersen AR, Lassen NA (1988) Cerebral blood flow by HMPAO/SPECT in senile dementias. In: Agnoli A, Cahn J, Lassen NA, Mayeux R (eds) Current problems in senile dementias. John Libbey, Paris, pp 399–408

Hemodynamic Subtypes of Dementia of the Alzheimer Type: Clinical and Neuropsychological Characteristics

P. Celsis, A. Agniel, M. Puel, J. F. Démonet, A. Rascol, and J. P. Marc-Vergnes

Summary

We studied 91 consecutive patients with probable Alzheimer's disease. From the cerebral blood flow (CBF) measurements obtained by single photon emission computer tomography (SPECT), three normalized indexes of asymmetry (Z-scores) were calculated for characterizing the patient's CBF pattern. Differences in the clinical and neuropsychological profiles of the hemodynamic subtypes thus defined were assessed. Twenty-nine patients presented with predominant posterior hypoperfusion, and ten with predominant anterior hypoperfusion. Forty-five patients exhibited a significant lateral asymmetry, 31 with preponderant left hemisphere defect and 14 with predominant right hypoperfusion. Thirteen patients demonstrated a particularly striking hypoperfusion of the deep subcortical regions but cortical CBF was not lower than that of controls. Nineteen patients presented with weak asymmetry, focal deficit or even normal pattern and were classified as borderline. Eighteen of the 28 patients examined twice did not modify their CBF pattern at second assessment; most of the 10 who did change had been ascribed first in the borderline, "buffer" group. Significant differences were observed in some of the clinical and neuropsychological features of subgroups. The posterior group showed higher global severity, higher right impairment and higher instrumental and memory deficits. In the anterior subgroup, left hemisphere impairment was severe and psychiatric disorders were more marked. In the subgroup with lateral asymmetry, there was a strong correlation between the CBF pattern and the side of predominant cognitive impairment. Age-of-onset was significantly higher in the subgroup with subcortical hypoperfusion, but the duration of disease did not differ; instrumental deficit was less pronounced but memory troubles were no less severe. In the borderline subgroup, age-of-onset was lower and dementia was far less severe, especially with regards to the instrumental deficit. Thus, a hemodynamic subtyping appears useful in assessing the heterogeneity of senile dementia of the Alzheimer type, all the more so as there is increasing evidence of the absolute necessity of integrating the model of heterogeneity regardless of the aim of the study.

Introduction

Most of the first studies on cerebral metabolism or blood flow in Alzheimer's disease using positron emission tomography (PET) pointed to bilateral, parietotemporal defects, which thus came to be considered the "classical" pattern of the disease (Frackowiak et al. 1981; Friedland et al. 1983; Foster et al. 1984; Cutler et al. 1985; Duara et al. 1986). Yet, in our experience, the existence of clearly different patterns became obvious soon after we proceeded to the first assessments of regional cerebral blood flow (CBF) in patients with clinically diagnosed dementia of the Alzheimer type (DAT). However, as flow abnormalities seemed to cluster in a limited number of consistent subtypes, we decided to assess the CBF profiles in a large series of almost 100 right-handed patients, and to study their relationships with some clinical and neuropsychological features. At the root of our work is the idea that, in the framework of the model of heterogeneity that is now largely accepted for DAT (Friedland et al. 1988; Riege and Metter 1988; Kaszniak 1988; Haxby et al. 1988), identifying hemodynamic subtypes with distinct clinical and neuropsychological profiles may help to improve our knowledge of the obviously complex dementing processes labeled as "dementia of the Alzheimer type."

Material and Methods

Patients

Out of a series of 114 consecutive patients referred to the Department of Neurology for presumptive Primary Degenerative Dementia (PDD) within a 4-year period, we retained 91 patients who met the DSM III criteria for PDD and the NINCDS-ADRDA criteria for probable Alzheimer's disease. Their Hachinski's ischemic scores were 4 or lower and none of the patients demonstrated a focal brain abnormality on computed tomography (CT) scan. In all cases, folic acid deficiency, hypothyroidism, tertiary neurosyphilis, pernicious anemia and alcohol abuse were ruled out. Table 1 gives the sex ratio, the mean and range of age, age-of-onset and duration of disease in our series of patients.

Controls

Thirty age-matched, normal volunteers were studied as controls (Table 1). They had a normal neurological examination, no history of cerebral vascular or psychiatric disease and a normal CT scan.

Informed consent was obtained from patients or their relatives and from volunteers.

Table 1. Sex ratio, age, age of onset and duration of disease in the groups of subjects

	Patients N=91		Controls N=30	
	Male	Female	Mean	Female
	36	55	15	15
	Mean	Range	Mean	Range
Age	68.3	52–87	62.7	52–75
Age-at-onset	65	50–84		
Duration	3.1	1–11		

Methods

Regional CBF was measured by SPECT and intravenous injection of xenon-133 in three transverse slices parallel and centered 1, 5 and 9 cm above the orbito-meatal plane. Quantitation of CBF was obtained using an algorithm previously described (Celsis et al. 1981). Large regions of interest were defined in the OM + 5 slice according to predefined templates (Fig. 1).

From the flow values obtained in the ROIs, normalized indexes of asymmetry were calculated according to the following formula: $IA = (A - mA)/sA$ with $A = 2 (F_1 - F_2)/(F_1 + F_2)$, where mA and sA are the mean and standard deviation of the weighted difference between the mean flows F_1 and F_2 observed in normals, in two selected regions or group of regions. Thus, these indexes are Z-scores expressed in units of control standard deviation.

By varying the selected regions, we obtained an index of anterior-posterior asymmetry ($F_1 = F_2$ and $F_2 = TP$ in both hemispheres; Fig. 1), of lateral asymmetry (F_1 = right hemisphere, F_2 = left hemisphere) and of cortical-subcortical asymmetry ($F_1 = F + I + TP$ and $F_2 = ASC + PSC$ for both sides; Fig. 1).

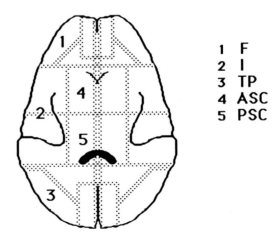

1 F
2 I
3 TP
4 ASC
5 PSC

Fig. 1. Regions of interest in the OM + 5 cm slice: *F*, frontal; *I*, insular; *TP*, temporoparietal; *ASC*, anterior subcortical; *PSC*, posterior subcortical

Asymmetries were considered significant when the index absolute value was higher than 2, with the site of the predominant hypoperfusion being determined according to the index sign.

Neuropsychological Evaluation

Extensive neuropsychological testing was administered to each patient to assess the cognitive deficit and the psychiatric disorders. Some subtests were varied according to the patient's mental status. Cortical functions were evaluated using the protocol MT 85 for language capacities, PEGV and Benton facial recognition test for visual gnosic activities, and Rey-Osterrieth complex figure, Bender gestalt test and WAIS block design subtest for constructive practical abilities. Memory troubles were assessed using the Wechsler memory scale, Benton visual retention test and 144 memory battery scale. Intellectual and operative abilities were evaluated through the WAIS arithmetic subtest and Raven progressive matrices. The Mini-Mental Score (MMS) was also used as an index of global severity [for references on neuropsychological tests, see Celsis et al. (1987)].

The existence and severity of psychiatric disorders were recorded from information obtained from the patient and/or provided by caregivers and derived from interviews and/or direct observation of behavior during hospitalization and/or from the evaluation of personality and behavioral changes through standardized scales such as the Hamilton Rating Scale for depression (Hamilton 1960) and the Blessed Dementia Scale (Blessed et al. 1968).

From the bulk of neuropsychological data thus obtained, the severity of the instrumental deficit (language, practical and gnosic activites) of the left and right hemisphere dysfunction (i.e., mainly language versus visuospatial deficit), of the memory impairment and of the psychiatric disorders was scored from 0 (absence) to 10 (extremely severe) by two trained, independent neuropsychologists blind to the flow data. Averaging the two scores provided five values that characterized the patient's neuropsychological status.

Results

Table 2 shows the number of patients in different subgroups defined according to the value of the indexes of hemodynamic asymmetry. It should be pointed out that the anterior, posterior and deep groups are mutually exclusive, as are obviously the left and right ones. However, anterior-posterior and cortical-subcortical asymmetries can be associated with a lateral asymmetry.

Twenty-nine patients, i.e., only 32%, showed a predominant hypoperfusion in the posterior association cortices. In 16 of them, there was no noticeable interhemispheric asymmetry. Figure 2 shows the flow map of one of these patients, which corresponds to the classical defects commonly described in DAT patients. In six patients, the posterior deficit largely predominated in the left hemisphere, involving a lateral asymmetry, such as for the patient shown in Fig. 3. In seven

Table 2. Sample size of the hemodynamic subtypes

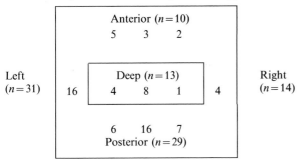

Borderline ($n=19$), Weak asymmetry ($n=12$), Focal ($n=3$),
Normal pattern ($n=4$)

cases, the posterior abnormality largely predominated in the right posterior cortex, as in Fig. 4.

Conversely, ten patients presented with predominant anterior hypoperfusion, showing a flow pattern such as that in Fig. 5. In half of the patients of this group, prominent left anterior hypoperfusion was observed, as in Fig. 6.

The third subtype we characterized by the flow pattern which corresponds to a group of 13 patients with preponderant deep, subcortical hypoperfusion, without any obvious defect in the cortical areas. Figure 7 shows an image of the flow pattern observed in one of these patients.

Sixteen patients had no anterior-posterior or cortical-subcortical asymmetry, but they showed a preponderant hypoperfusion of the left hemisphere, as in the case in Fig. 8.

Similarly, four patients showed a predominant right hypoperfusion not associated with another striking asymmetry, as can be observed for the patient shown in Fig. 9.

Finally, 19 patients did not meet our quantitative criteria for hemodynamic asymmetry. Since most of them presented with a weak asymmetry (index absolute value lower than 2) or with a focal defect such as those we described previously that were associated with a selective cognitive deficit (Celsis et al. 1987), we called this group "borderline." However, four patients of this group did exhibit a flow distribution that could not be distinguished from that of normal subjects, as in the patient shown in Fig. 10, who was still undoubtedly demented at the date of examination, with a MMS score equal to 17 4 years after onset.

Lastly, it is noteworthy that half of the patients demonstrated marked interhemispheric asymmetry, with the hypoperfusion predominating in the left hemisphere in two-thirds of the cases (31 versus only 14 for right hemisphere).

The temporal stability of our hemodynamic patterns proved to be good for the definite subtypes, as were the metabolic patterns of the patients studied by Grady et al. (1986). Indeed, the first results of a longitudinal survey still in progress indicate that, for 18 of the 28 patients who were examined at least twice, there was no change in subgrouping. Figure 11 shows, for example, the successive flow maps of a patient of the posterior group, demonstrating the consistency of the flow pattern within a 3-year period. By contrast, seven of the ten patients who changed were first ascribed to the "borderline" subtype. This subtype thus appears as a buffer, from which patients will distribute into definite groups with progression of the disease and worsening of flow defects, as was seen in one patient who moved from focal, borderline abnormality (Fig. 12) to clear-cut, whole left hemisphere hypoperfusion (Fig. 13).

The hemodynamic subtypes we have defined above were found to present some differences in their clinical and neuropsychological profiles.

First, there were significant relationships between cognitive and hemodynamic lateral asymmetries. As shown in Table 3, left hemisphere predominant hypoperfusion was associated with more severe left hemisphere dysfunction, and, conversely, preponderant right hypoperfusion was accompanied by marked right cognitive dysfunction. Moreover, the correlation between the difference in left-right dysfunction and the index of lateral hemodynamic asymmetry was highly significant (Table 3). These results are in agreement with those previously reported by authors using PET (Friedland et al. 1985; Haxby et al. 1985).

Table 4 gives the sex ratio, mean age-of-onset and mean duration of disease in the posterior, anterior, deep and borderline subgroups. The deep subtype mainly includes females (11 of 13). Mean age-at-onset is significantly higher in

Table 3. Relations between cognitive and hemodynamic lateral asymmetries. Correlation between cognitive lateral asymmetry (left hemisphere dysfunction score — right hemisphere dysfunction score) and the index of hemodynamic lateral asymmetry: $r = 0.59$, df $= 89$, $p < 0.0001$

Cognitive dysfunction score	Side of preponderant hypoperfusion			
	Left	No asymmetry	Right	
	($n = 31$)	($n = 46$)	($n = 14$)	
Left hemisphere	4.5	3.1	3.4	$p < 0.05$
Right hemisphere	3.0	3.2	4.9	$p < 0.05$

Table 4. Clinical data and mean CBF in hemodynamic subtypes

	Posterior ($n = 29$)	Anterior ($n = 10$)	Deep ($n = 13$)	Borderline ($n = 19$)	
Sex ratio (M/F)	17/12	3/7	2/11	5/14	
Age-at-onset	63	67.5	71.3	61.4	$p < 0.05$
Duration (years)	3.6	1.8	2.6	3.1	
Mean CBF (ml/100 g per minute)	45.9	48.2	56.1	47.5	$p < 0.05$

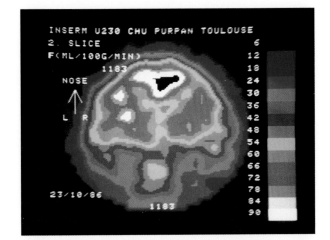

Fig. 2. Flow map (ml/100 g per minute, OM + 5) of a patient with the classical pattern of Alzheimer's disease, i.e., a bilateral posterior hypoperfusion

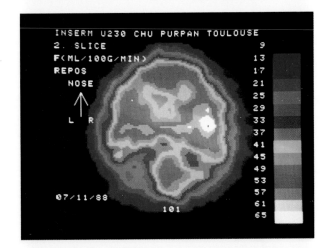

Fig. 3. Flow map (ml/100 g per minute, OM + 5) of a patient with left posterior hypoperfusion

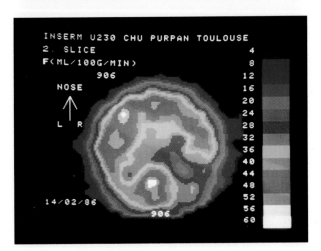

Fig. 4. Flow map (ml/100 g per minute, OM + 5) of a patient with right posterior hypoperfusion

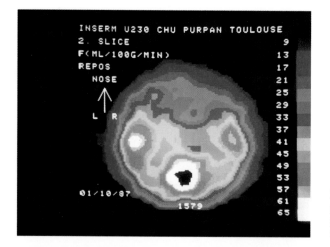

Fig. 5. Flow map (ml/100 g per minute, OM + 5) of a patient with bilateral anterior hypoperfusion

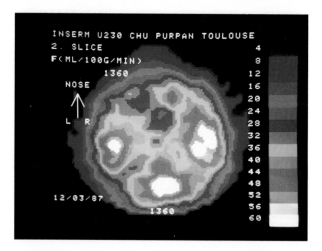

Fig. 6. Flow map (ml/100 g per minute, OM + 5) of a patient with left anterior hypoperfusion

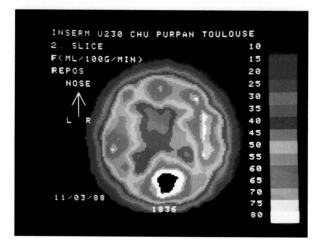

Fig. 7. Flow map (ml/100 g per minute, OM + 5) of a patient with deep, subcortical hypoperfusion

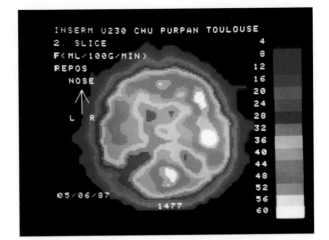

Fig. 8. Flow map (ml/100 g per minute, OM + 5) of a patient with predominant hypoperfusion of the whole left hemisphere

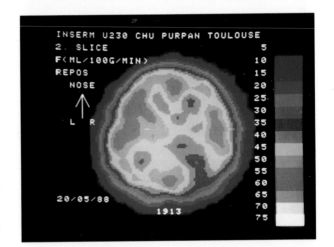

Fig. 9. Flow map (ml/100 g per minute, OM + 5) of a patient with predominant hypoperfusion of the whole right hemisphere

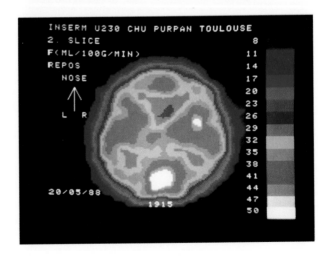

Fig. 10. Flow map (ml/ 100 g per minute, OM + 5) of a patient with normal pattern

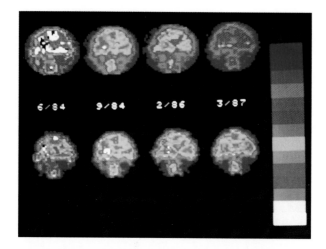

Fig. 11. Successive flow maps obtained in a patient of the posterior group within a period of three years, showing the temporal stability of the pattern. *Top row*, absolute flow values; *bottom row*, pixel to mean slice values

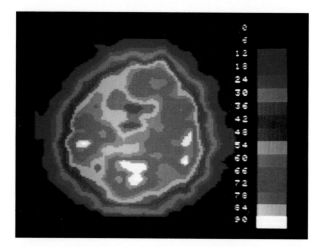

Fig. 12. Flow map (ml/100 g per minute, OM + 5) of a patient with focal, left anterior hypoperfusion

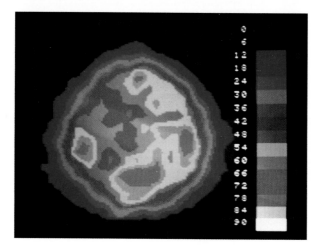

Fig. 13. Flow map (ml/100 g per minute, OM + 5) of the same patient as in Fig. 12 (color scale unchanged), showing the progression of the flow defect 22 months after the first measurement

this subgroup, and these patients have late-onset dementia. Duration of disease does not differ significantly between groups, although it tends to be shorter in the anterior group.

It is also interesting to note that mean CBF in the deep group is not decreased (Table 4); on the average, whole CBF is almost identical to that measured in age- and sex-matched controls. This means that patients of this group have no, or only very mild, flow defect in the neocortex.

Table 5 shows that there is a significant difference between the mean MMS scores of the subgroups, with dementia being less severe in the borderline group, and, to a lesser degree, in the deep group, whereas overall severity does not differ between the posterior and anterior subtypes. Accordingly, the instrumental deficit (i.e., the impairment of language, practical and gnosic activities) is less severe in the deep and borderline groups, whereas it is of comparable magnitude in the posterior and anterior ones. Yet it should be noted that, although quantitatively comparable in these last two groups, the instrumental deficit does differ qualitatively: left dysfunction is much more pronounced than right dysfunction in the anterior group (5.5 vs. 3.6), owing to the preponderance of language deficit of the nonfluent type, while right dysfunction slightly predominates in the posterior group (4.8 vs. 4.1), where visuospatial defects and apraxia appear more severe than the language disturbance of the fluent, posterior type.

By contrast, no significant difference was found in the severity of memory impairment and psychiatric disorders (Table 5), although memory troubles predominate slightly in the posterior group and psychiatric disorders in the anterior one.

Group discrepancies in instrumental deficit versus memory troubles and psychiatric disorders are further illustrated in the last two lines of Table 5, which shows the difference between the instrumental score and the memory or psychiatric scores. Psychiatric disorders thus appear disproportionately severe compared to instrumental deficit in patients of the deep group and, to a lesser degree, in borderline patients. Similarly, memory impairment is relatively more pronounced in the deep and borderline subtypes.

Table 5. Neuropsychological data in hemodynamic subtypes

	Posterior ($n=29$)	Anterior ($n=10$)	Deep ($n=13$)	Borderline ($n=19$)	
MMS	13.8	13.6	16.5	22.0	$p<0.01$
Instrumental deficit	5.6	5.4	3.8	3.6	$p<0.01$
Memory troubles	5.5	5.0	4.6	4.6	
Psychiatric disorders	3.2	4.0	3.8	2.7	
Difference instrumental− psychiatrie	2.4	1.4	0.0	0.8	$p<10^{-3}$
Difference instrumental− memory	0.1	0.4	−0.8	−1.0	$p<0.05$

Conclusion

In conclusion, our study of a large series of almost 100 consecutive patients shows that consistent CBF patterns can be recognized that allow hemodynamic subtyping of DAT. Furthermore, differences in the clinical and neuropsychological characteristics associated with these subtypes have been demonstrated, with good concordance between flow defects and cognitive deficits. These results confirm and reinforce the notion of heterogeneity in DAT, a notion that should be kept in mind, regardless of the type of study. They can serve, for instance, as guidelines for neuropathological and neurochemical studies or even therapeutic trials.

In addition, a particularly interesting finding, in our opinion, is that of a peculiar subtype of DAT characterized by a hypoperfusion of the deep regions associated with late-onset and predominance of memory troubles and psychiatric disorders. This subtype may correspond to the patients with late-onset, recently reported by Zubenko et al. (1989), who demonstrate a relative sparing of the neocortex with regards to specific neuropathological and neurochemical deficits. It may be, therefore, that the old distinction between senile and presenile dementia deserves new consideration.

Acknowledgements. The authors thank G. Viallard for invaluable help in processing the data and Mrs. T. Pujol and C. Blanchard for technical assistance and management of patients and volunteers.

References

Blessed G, Tomlinson B, Roth M (1968) The association between quantitative measures of dementia and of senile change in the cerebral grey matter of elderly subjects. Brit J Psychiat 114:797–811

Celsis P, Goldman T, Henriksen L, Lassen NA (1981) A method for calculating regional cerebral blood flow from emission computed tomography of inert gas concentrations. J Comput Assist Tomogr 5:641–645

Celsis P, Agniel A, Puel M, Rascol A, Marc-Vergnes JP (1987) Focal cerebral hypoperfusion and selective cognitive deficit in dementia of the Alzheimer type. J Neurol Neurosurg Psychiatry 50:1602–1612

Cutler NR, Haxby JV, Duara R, Grady CL, Kay AD, Kessler RM, Sundaram M, Rapoport SI (1985) Clinical history, brain metabolism, and neuropsychological function in Alzheimer's disease. Ann Neurol 18:298–309

Duara R, Grady C, Haxby J, Sundaram M, Cutler NR, Heston L, Moore A, Schlageter N, Larson S, Rapoport SI (1986) Positron emission tomography in Alzheimer's disease. Neurology 36:879–887

Foster NL, Chase TN, Mansi L, Brooks R, Fedio P, Patronas NJ, Di Chiro G (1984) Cortical abnormalities in Alzheimer's disease. Ann Neurol 16:649–654

Frackowiak RS, Pozzilli C, Legg NJ, Du Boulay GH, Marshall J, Lenzi GL, Jones T (1981) Regional cerebral oxygen supply and utilization in dementia, a clinical and physiological study with oxygen-15 and positron tomography. Brain 104:753–778

Friedland RP, Budinger TF, Ganz E, Yano Y, Mathis CA, Koss B, Ober BA, Huesman RH, Derenzo SE (1983) Regional cerebral metabolic alterations in dementia of the Alzheimer type: positron emission tomography with [^{18}F]fluorodeoxyglucose. J Comput Assist Tomogr 7:590–598

Friedland RF, Budinger TF, Koss E, Ober BA (1985) Alzheimer's disease: anterior-posterior and lateral hemispheric alterations in cortical glucose utilization. Neurosci Lett 53:235–240

Friedland RP, Koss E, Haxby JV, Grady CL, Luxenberg J, Schapiro MB, Kaye J (1988) Alzheimer's disease: clinical and biological heterogeneity. Ann Intern Med 109:298–311

Grady CL, Haxby JV, Schlageter NL, Berg G, Rapoport SI (1986) Stability of metabolic and neuropsychological asymmetries in dementia of the Alzheimer type. Neurology 36:1390–1392

Hamilton M (1960) A rating scale for depression. J Neurol Neurosurg Psychiat 23:56–62

Haxby JV, Duara R, Grady CL, Cutler NR, Rapoport SI (1985) Relations between neuropsychological and cerebral metabolic asymmetries in early Alzheimer's disease. J Cereb Blood Flow Metabol 5:193–200

Haxby JV, Grady CL, Koss E, Horwitz B, Schapiro M, Friedland RP, Rapoport SI (1988) Heterogeneous anterior-posterior metabolic patterns in dementia of the Alzheimer type. Neurology 38:1853–1863

Kaszniak AW (1988) Cognition in Alzheimer's disease: theoretic models and clinical implications. Neurobiol Aging 9:92–94

Riege WH, Metter EJ (1988) Cognitive and brain imaging measures of Alzheimer's disease. Neurobiol Aging 9:69–86

Zubenko GS, Moossy J, Martinez AJ, Rao GR, Kopp U, Hanin I (1989) A brain regional analysis of morphologic and cholinergic abnormalities in Alzheimer's disease. Arch Neurol 46:634–638

Nuclear Magnetic Resonance Study
of Phospholipid Metabolites in Alzheimer's Disease

J. W. Pettegrew and W. E. Klunk

Summary

In summary, both postmortem and antemortem studies demonstrate that the levels of PME are elevated in the brains of AD patients. Similar levels of PME are found normally in the developing brain. It is truly remarkable that a devastating disease like AD should resemble the normal developing brain at a metabolic/molecular level. The PME elevations appear to be an early molecular alteration in AD and can now be assessed antemortem with in vivo ^{31}P NMR spectroscopy. This will prove invaluable in following the metabolic progression of the disease, will provide insights which can be used to develop new pharmacological treatments and will allow the metabolic response to pharmacological intervention to be assessed noninvasively.

The findings of antemortem alterations of erythrocyte membrane molecular dynamics and Na^+-Li^+ biology in AD patients will also provide valuable new insights into the molecular pathophysiology of AD. In addition, these studies require only a finger prick of blood (5 µl) and, therefore, can be used to study large populations of patients. Although the final chapters of AD are yet to be written, there are now significant insights into the "molecular plot."

Introduction

Alzheimer's disease (AD) is a devastating disorder manifested by progressive loss of memory and decline in other cognitive functions. The diagnostic hallmarks of AD are increased numbers of senile plaques (SP) and neurofibrillary tangles (NFT) in the cerebral cortex as compared to age-matched controls. However, these morphological findings are not specific to AD and could represent end-stage markers of the disease process. Therefore, the study of SP and NFT might not provide insights into the fundamental, initial molecular events that cause the disease. The morphological markers do, however, provide a time scale for measuring the disease progression, since presumably the greater the numbers of SP and NFT, the longer the disease has been present. From this point of view, SP and NFT can be used for correlations with measures of metabolic and molecular alterations observed in autopsy brain. In particular, metabolic or molecular alterations that appear to occur prior to the occurrence of significant numbers of SP or NFT could represent earlier and possibly more fundamental alterations in AD than the morphological markers.

Phosphomonoesters and Phosphodiesters

In vitro ^{31}P nuclear magnetic resonance (NMR) studies reveal alterations in membrane phospholipid metabolism in AD autopsy- and biopsy-derived brain tissue (Pettegrew et al. 1984 a, 1987 a and d, 1988 b, 1989 d). Elevated levels of phosphomonoesters (PME) are inversely correlated with the numbers of SP; there is no correlation with the numbers of NFT (Pettegrew et al. 1988 d). PME are precursors of membrane phospholipids as well as products of phospholipase C and phosphodiesterase activities and are normally found in high levels in developing brain (Pettegrew et al. 1989 c). From this perspective AD brain resembles developing brain. Since the levels of PME are inversely correlated with the numbers of SP, the molecular alterations giving rise to the PME probably antedate the increase in SP numbers. Phosphodiester (PDE) levels in AD brain have a positive correlation with the numbers of SP and no correlation with the numbers of NFT (Pettegrew et al. 1988 d). PDE are breakdown products of membrane phospholipids due to phospholipase A activity, and elevated levels of PDE are found in normal aging and in brain degeneration (Pettegrew et al. 1989 c). Since the PDE are positively correlated with the numbers of SP, both probably reflect degenerative processes occurring later in the course of the disease.

The PME have striking conformational similarities with L-glutamate and N-methyl-D-aspartate (Pettegrew et al. 1988 b) and alter the population excitatory postsynaptic potentials (EPSP) of CA1 pyramidal cells in the hippocampus (Barrionuevo et al. 1988; Pettegrew et al. 1988 c; Bradler et al., submitted). The PME phosphoethanolamine and L-phosphoserine depress the amplitude of the EPSP in a dose-dependent fashion (10 μM – 1.0 mM). In contrast, the PME phosphocholine depresses at low concentration (10 μm) but markedly increases the EPSP amplitude at higher concentrations (1 mM). The concentrations of PME in AD brain are as high as 5–7 mM. This is the same concentration range of PME as found in normal developing brain (Pettegrew et al. 1987 a). These findings suggest that the PME could depress L-glutamate-mediated neurotransmission at lower concentrations and thereby contribute to memory problems typical of AD. However, at higher concentrations, phosphocholine could act as an excitatory neurotoxin and target neurons with L-glutamate receptors, such as large pyramidal neuron, for cell death. This provides a possible explanation for the prominent memory loss early in AD and the predominance of neuropathology in large pyramidal neurons.

The PME and PDE are also very "membrane active" molecules. The PME induce dose-dependent changes in membrane molecular dynamics of normal human erythrocytes and platelets (Pettegrew et al. 1989 a). In fact, the recent observations of altered platelet membrane "fluidity" in AD patients by Zubenko and coworkers (1984, 1987 a and b) can be reproduced in normal human platelets after brief (30 min) incubation with the PME and PDE. Likewise, similar alterations in erythrocyte membrane molecular dynamics can be produced after brief incubation with the PME and PDE (Pettegrew et al. 1989 a).

The PME, but not the PDE, also alter the phase and conformation of synthetic model membranes (Pettegrew 1989 a and b; Panchalingam and Pettegrew 1989; Pettegrew and Panchalingam 1989). Model membranes composed of the phospholipids phosphatidylethanolamine (PtdE) and phosphatidylserine (PtdS), but not phosphatidylcholine (PtdC), are altered by the PME. PtdE and PtdS are predominantly located on the cytoplasmic face of plasma membranes. The PME change the model membranes from a normal bilayer phase to micellar and hexagonal II phases. The micellar phase is normally found in vesicles such as those which contain neurotransmitter molecules packaged for release. The hexagonal II phase is the phase that promotes the fusion of vesicles to bilayers and, thereby, promotes the transport of vesicles across bilayer membranes. These findings taken together provide a molecular mechanism whereby the PME could induce their own packaging into vesicles and then promote the release of the vesicles from neurons. Of course, other neurotransmitters could also be packaged and released by the same PME-induced mechanisms.

Membrane Phospholipids

The phospholipids PtdC, PtdE, and PtdS are all decreased in AD brain compared to non-AD demented controls (Pettegrew et al. 1988 a). Both PtdE and PtdS are inversely correlated with the numbers of SP, with no NFT correlation. PtdC has a nonlinear correlation with the numbers of SP, which increases up to approximately 10 SP/200 magnification and then decreases (Pettegrew et al. 1989 b). This suggests increased synthesis of PtdC early in the disease which could shunt available choline away from acetylcholine synthesis, resulting in a hypocholinergic state (Pettegrew 1989 a and b).

Phospholipid Enzymes

Recent studies in collaboration with Julian Kanfer in Winnepeg have investigated the activity in several enzymes involved in phospholipid metabolism. These studies were conducted on samples obtained from AD brain and non-AD demented control brains. Choline acetyltransferase activity is decreased in AD brain ($p=0.001$); the activity correlates inversely withn the numbers of SP ($p=0.05$, $R^2=0.7$), with no NFT correlation. Choline kinase activity is also decreased in AD brain ($p=0.0001$) and correlates inversely with the number of SP ($p=0.08$, $R^2=0.7$), with no NFT correlation. Measures of glycerol phosphodiesterase activity, however, reveal increased amounts of phosphocholine released in AD brain ($p=0.01$), without differences in the amounts of choline released. The amount of phosphocholine released does not appear to correlate with the numbers of SP or NFT. The activities of phospholipase D and A_2 are unchanged in AD brain and there is no correlation with the numbers of SP or NFT.

In Vivo Brain Studies

In vivo antemortem ^{31}P NMR studies of AD patients confirm the increased brain levels of PME as compared to age-matched normal controls and demented patients with multiple subcortical infarcts (Gdowski et al. 1988; Brown et al. 1989). Further in vivo ^{31}P NMR studies suggest that the PME do not correlate with the Mattis dementia scores (Pettegrew et al., unpublished results). However, the levels of PDE are inversely correlated with the Mattis scores and the levels of phosphocreatine (PCr) are positively correlated with the Mattis scores. The intracellular pH (Pettegrew et al. 1988e) is normal. These findings are in keeping with the in vitro findings and again suggest that the elevated PME reflect an early event in the pathogenesis of AD. In contrast the dementia appears to reflect the degeneration of neuritic processes giving rise to increased PDE. The phosphocreatine-Mattis correlation suggests either decreased synthesis or increased utilization of PCr with disease progression. With a normal intracellular pH, the PCr findings are not explainable by a shift in the creatine kinase equilibrium. Since studies in rats demonstrate an inverse correlation between the levels of PME and PCr after brief hypoxia (Pettegrew et al., unpublished results), the role of cellular hypoxia in AD needs to be re-examined.

In Vivo Erythrocyte Studies

Since the PME and PDE are so membrane active, they could be released from brain cells, cross the blood-brain barrier and enter the general circulation. The PME could also potentially be produced in other organs in AD, such as the liver, and enter the general circulation from these sites. Once in the general circulation, the PME and PDE could insert themselves into the membranes of circulating cells such as the erythrocyte or the platelet or into fibroblasts.

Recently this latter possibility was investigated by measuring membrane molecular dynamics in erythrocytes obtained from probable AD patients (ADRDA-NINCDS criteria) and normal controls. The erythrocyte was chosen for study because the circulating erythrocyte contains only one membrane, the plasma membrane, and, therefore, one can be certain that any demonstrated membrane alterations are coming from the plasma membrane and not from the endoplasmic reticulum, mitochondria or nuclear membranes. Also, the mature circulating human erythrocyte does not synthesize membrane lipids after the reticulocyte stage. Instead, the erythrocyte membrane phospholipids, cholesterol and fatty acids undergo exchange transfer with circulating lipids and lipoproteins. Because of this, the erythrocyte can be considered a potential "reporter cell" for lipid alterations occurring in the CNS or other organs.

Previous studies have provided evidence for alterations in erythrocyte membranes in AD. These alterations include:

1) altered molecular organization of erythrocyte cytoskeletal proteins without alterations in the molecular dynamics of the superficial hydrocarbon layer of the membrane, Na^+-K^+ ATPase or acetylcholinesterase activities, SDS-polyacrylamide electrophoresis of the membrane proteins (Markesbery et al. 1980) or the motion of erythrocyte surface sialic acid groups (Butterfield et al. 1985);
2) increased choline efflux rate across the erythrocyte membrane (Butterfield et al. 1985; Blass et al. 1985; Sherman et al. 1986);
3) increased Na^+-Li^+ countertransport (Diamond et al. 1983);
4) increased erythrocyte choline; and
5) decreased erythrocyte membrane PdtC (Miller et al. 1989).

To date, we have investigated membrane molecular dynamics in five probable AD cases and six normal controls (Pettegrew et al., unpublished results). In addition, Na^+ and Li^+ membrane transport and intracellular biology were studied in five probable AD cases and five controls (Pettegrew and Panchalingam, unpublished results). The studies of membrane molecular dynamics reveal increased molecular motion in the hydrocarbon core of probable AD erythrocytes compared to controls ($p=0.02$). Thee findings are virtually identical to those observed in AD platelets by Zubenko and coworkers (1984, 1987a and b) and also those induced in normal control erythrocytes after incubation with the PME (Pettegrew et al. 1989a). The increased membrane molecular dynamics is the opposite of what is observed with normal aging, in which there is a decrease in membrane molecular dynamics. Increased membrane molecular dynamics is observed in normal fetal and immature tissues and supports the observation that the PME are normally high in developing brain and paradoxically elevated in AD brain.

To determine if altered membrane molecular dynamics in AD erythrocytes could alter Na^+, Li^+ transport or intracellular binding, ^{23}Na and ^7Li NMR studies were conducted. The theory and application of ^{23}Na and ^7Li NMR to human erythrocytes have previously been reported (Pettegrew et al. 1984b, 1987b and c; Pettegrew and Woessner 1989). These preliminary studies reveal that the Li^+ entry/efflux ratio and the intracellular Li^+ rotational mobility ($p=0.0006$) are altered in AD erythrocytes. In this small sample, no alterations were observed in Li^+ translational mobility or either the rotational or translational mobilities of Na^+. The Li^+ alterations could potentially contribute to the increased toxicity of Li^+ which has been observed in AD patients (Pomara et al. 1984; Kelwala et al. 1984) and the altered Li^+-Na^+ countertransport also noted in AD erythrocytes (Diamond et al. 1983).

References

Barrionuevo G, Bradler JE, Pettegrew JW (1988) Electrophysiological effects of phosphomonoesters on hippocampal brain slices (Abstract). Neurology 38 (Suppl 1):336

Blass JP, Hanin I, Barclay L, Kopp U, Reding MJ (1985) Red blood cell abnormalities in Alzheimer disease. J Am Geriatric Soc 33:401–405

Brown GG, Levine SR, Gorell JM, Pettegrew JW, Gdowski JW, Bueri JA, Helpern JA, Welch KMA (1989) In vivo ^{31}P NMR profiles of Alzheimer's disease and multiple subcortical infarct dementia. Neurology, in press

Butterfield DA, Farmer BT, II Markesbery WR (1985) Alzheimer's disease: no alteration in the physical state of erythrocyte membrane glycoconugates. Ann Neurol 18:104–105

Diamond JM, Matsuyama SS, Meier K, Jarvik LF (1983) Elevation of erythrocyte countertransport rates in Alzheimer's dementia. N Engl J Med 309:1061–1062

Gdowski JW, Brown GG, Levine SR, Smith M, Helpern J, Bueri J, Gorell J, Welch KMA (1988) Patterns of phospholipid metabolism differ between Alzheimer and multi-infarct dementia (Abstract). Neurology 38 (Suppl 1):268

Kelwala S, Pomara N, Stanley M, Sitaram N, Gershon S (1984) Lithium-induced accentuation of extrapyramidal symptoms in individuals with Alzheimer's disease. J Clin Psychiat 45:343–344

Markesbery WR, Leung PK, Butterfield DA (1980) Spin label and biochemical studies of erythrocyte membranes in Alzheimer's disease. J Neurol Sci 45:323–330

Miller BL, Jenden D, Tang C, Read S (1989) Choline and choline-bound phospholipids in aging and Alzheimer's disease. Neurology 39 (Suppl 1):254

Panchalingam K, Pettegrew JW (1989) Evidence of Al^{3+} and phosphomonoester interaction with model membranes. Bull Magn Reson, in press

Pettegrew JW (1989a) Molecular insights into Alzheimer's disease. NY Acad Sci, in press

Pettegrew JW (1989b) Molecular insights into Alzheimer's disease. In: Boller F, Katzman R, Rascol A, Signoret JL, Christen Y (eds) The biological markers of Alzheimer's disease. Heidelberg, Springer, pp 83–104

Pettegrew JW, Panchalingam K (1989) Solid state ^{31}P and ^{27}Al NMR studies of model membranes and mammalian brain: possible implications for Alzheimer's disease. In: Pettegrew JW (ed) Nuclear magnetic resonance: the principles and applications of NMR spectroscopy and imaging to biomedical research. New York, Springer, in press

Pettegrew JW, Kopp SJ, Minshew NJ, Glonek T, Feliksik JM, Tow JP, Cohen MM (1987a) ^{31}P Nuclear magnetic resonance studies of phosphoglyceride metabolism in developing and degenerating brain: preliminary observations. J Neuropathol Exp Neurol 46:419–430

Pettegrew JW, McKeag D, Strychor S (1989a) Metabolites altered in Alzheimer's brain alter membrane properties. Soc Neurosci Abst 15:1110

Pettegrew JW, Minshew NJ, Cohen MM, Kopp SJ, Glonek T (1984a) P-31 NMR changes in Alzheimer's and Huntington's disease brain (Abstract). Neurology 34(1):281

Pettegrew JW, Moossy J, Panchalingam K, et al. (1989b) Correlation of phospholipids and senile plaques in Alzheimer's brain (Abstract). Neurology 39(1):396

Pettegrew JW, Moossy J, Strychor S, McKeag D, Boller F (1988a) Membrane phospholipid alterations in Alzheimer's brain (Abstract). Neurology 38:267

Pettegrew JW, Moossy J, Withers G, McKeag D, Panchalingam K (1988b) ^{31}P Nuclear magnetic resonance study of the brain in Alzheimer's disease. J Neuropath Exp Neurol 47(3):235–248

Pettegrew JW, Panchalingam K, McKeag D, Barrionuevo G (1988c) Metabolic effects of phosphomonoesters on hippocampal brain slices (Abstract). Neurology 28(1):323

Pettegrew JW, Panchalingam K, Moossy J, Martinez JA, Rao G, Boller F (1988d) Correlation of ^{31}P NMR and morphological findings in Alzheimer's disease. Arch Neurol 45:1093–1096

Pettegrew JW, Panchalingam K, Withers G, McKeag D, Strychor S (1989c) Changes in brain energy and phospholipid metabolism during development and aging in the Fischer 344 rat. J Neuropath Exp Neurol, in press

Pettegrew JW, Post JEM, Panchalingam K, Withers G, Woessner DE (1987b) ^{7}Li NMR study of normal human erythrocytes. J Magn Reson 71:504–519

Pettegrew JW, Short JE, Woessner RD, Strychor S, McKeag D, Armstrong J, Minshew NJ, Rush AJ (1987c) The effect of lithium on the membrane molecular dynamics of normal human erythrocytes. Biol Psych 2:857–871

Pettegrew JW, Withers G, Panchalingam K (1989d) ^{31}P NMR of brain aging and Alzheimer's disease. In: Pettegrew JW (ed) Nuclear magnetic resonance: the principles and applications of NMR spectroscopy and imaging to biomedical research. Springer, Berlin Heidelberg New York, in press

Pettegrew JW, Withers G, Panchalingam K, Post JEM (1988e) Considerations for brain pH assessment by ^{31}P NMR. Magn Reson Imaging 6:135–142

Pettegrew JW, Withers G, Panchalingam K, Post JFM (1987d) ^{31}P Nuclear magnetic resonance (NMR) spectrocopy of brain in aging and Alzheimer's disease. In: Wurtman RJ, Corkin SH, Growden JH (eds) Alzheimer's disease: advances in basic research and therapies. Center for Brain Sciences and Metabolism Charitable Trust, Cambridge, MA, pp 57–68

Pettegrew JW, Woessner D (1989) ^{23}Na and ^{7}Li NMR studies of mammalian cells: assessment of cation transport and cytoskeletal structure with application to manic depressive disease. In: Pettegrew JW (ed) Nuclear magnetic resonance: the principles and applications of NMR spectroscopy and imaging to biomedical research. Springer, Berlin Heidelberg New York, in press

Pettegrew JW, Woessner DE, Minshew NJ, Glonek T (1984b) Sodium-23 NMR analysis of human whole blood, erythrocytes, and plasma. Chemical shift, spin relaxation and intracellular sodium concentration studies. J Magn Reson 57:185–196

Pomara N, Block R, Domino E, Gershon S (1984) Decay in plasma lithium and normalization in red blood cell choline following cessation of lithium treatment in two elderly individuals with Alzheimer-type dementia. Biol Psych 19:919–922

Sherman KA, Gibson GE, Blass JP (1986) Human red blood cell choline uptake with age and Alzheimer's disesae. Neurobiol Aging 7:205–209

Zubenko GS, Cohen BM, Growdin J, Corkin S (1984) Cell membrane abnormality in Alzheimer's disease (Letter). Lancet II:235

Zubenko GS, Cohen BM, Reynolds CF, Boller F, Malinakova I, Keefe MA (1987a) Platelet membrane fluidity in Alzheimer's disease and major depression. Am J Psych 144:860–868

Zubenko GS, Malinakova I, Chojnacki B (1987b) Proliferation of internal membranes in platelets from patients with Alzheimer's disease. J Neuropathol Exp Neurol 46:407–418

Summary Comments on Presentations

S. I. Rapoport

When I became involved with Alzheimer's disease about 10 years ago, I and others thought it to be a global dementia – showing global changes in neuropathology, cognition, and brain metabolism. In the meantime, however, we have discovered that it is a much more subtle disease, and that it deserves to be examined in terms of the topography of the anatomical, functional, and neurochemical systems that it selectively affects. In my introductory paper, I posed the hypothesis that association brain areas (neocortical assocation areas as well as nonneocortical, phylogenically older regions that are connected with association neocortical areas) are more vulnerable to Alzheimer's disease than are other brain regions. This principle of selective regional vulnerability also applies, with different areas being affected, to Huntington's disease, Parkinson's disease, Pick's disease, and several other neurodegenerative disorders.

The consensus of this symposium is that the hypothesis of regional vulnerability in Alzheimer's disease is indeed quite reasonable. It is supported by in vivo and postmortem studies obtained with a variety of techniques. The hypothesis suggests, furthermore, that future research should be directed to discovering what makes certain brain regions vulnerable, using approaches such as immunocytochemistry and molecular biology and conducting comparative studies among primates. These approaches should bring us into contact with the genetics of Alzheimer's disease and perhaps suggest genes whose expression in vulnerable regions relates to the disease mechanism. For example, the growth-associated protein GAP-43 and the amyloid precursor protein, which contains a protease inhibitor, are found preferentially in association brain areas (Neve et al. 1988 a, b). Understanding their topographical distribution may provide an insight into the cause of Alzheimer's disease.

As regards neuropathology within the association neocortices, Dr. Morrison reported that only certain neurons are critically affected – pyramidal neurons of layer III and to some extent those of layer V. These neurons subserve long intracerebral cortico-cortical connections, and their pathology may result in a cortical disconnection syndrome underlying much of Alzheimer dementia. In the nondiseased brain, the vulnerable neurons can be identified by a marker antibody, SMI-32, raised against 168-kDa and 200-kDa subunits of neurofilament proteins, suggesting that phosphorylation of cytoskeletal proteins is defective in Alzheimer's disease.

Dr. Bowen's observation that glutamatergic markers are abnormal in the Alzheimer brain is consistent with Dr. Morrison's observations, as L-glutamate is

the major neurotransmitter of neurons which originate long cortico-cortical connections. Dr. Bowen's study also suggests that future drug trials be directed to
glutamatergic dysfunction in Alzheimer's disease.

The report by Drs. Hauw and Duyckaerts argues that cortical atrophy in the
Alzheimer brain results from dropout of vertically oriented cortical columns,
which are the fundamental building blocks of the mammalian neocortex. However, we are left with the dilemma of trying to relate Dr. Morrison's description of
a horizontal pathology and dropout of pyramidal neurons in layers III and V of
the neocortex with Dr. Hauw's suggestion of a transcortical, vertical pathology
involving all six layers. Dr. Hauw also noted that several nonneocortical regions
are pathological as well. My reading of the literature and my understanding of
Dr. Hauw's presentation is that nonneocortical pathology is neither indiscrimi-
nate nor global. The nucleus basalis of Meynert, the dorsal raphe nucleus, and
locus coeruleus neurons which frequently are lost in Alzheimer's disease provide
cholinergic, serotonergic, and noradrenergic innervation, respectively, to much of
the neocortex. In Alzheimer's disease, furthermore, the amygdaloid complex is
only selectively involved (newer more than older nuclei), as is the hippocampal
formation. From the report by Hyman et al. (1984) it appears likely that pathology of the entorhinal cortex disconnects the hippocampal formation from the
neocortex.

Although nonneocortical regions which are pathological in Alzheimer's disease are, for the most part, directly connected with the association neocortices,
some exceptions exist which at present are difficult to explain. Pathology of the
phylogenically older olfactory bulb (which, however, is connected with the amygdaloid formation) and of the retina remains to be understood.

Dr. Creasey showed that quantitative computer-assisted tomography (CT)
demonstrates accelerated ventricular dilatation in Alzheimer's disease and thus
can be used for the early diagnosis of Alzheimer's disease as a progressive organic
dementia. Her study clearly shows that cell loss occurs very early in the course of
Alzheimer's disease, even in mildly demented patients. Consequently, if pharma-
cotherapy is to be instituted, it should be initiated early, when as many neurons
as possible are still present, rather than late in the disease. Dr. Creasey emphasized the need to develop better techniques for the early diagnosis of Alzheimer's
disease, including serial, quantitative magnetic resonance imaging (MRI).

Dr. Leys pointed out that subcortical white matter lesions on CT (leukoaraiosis) in Alzheimer patients correlate with the density of neurofibrillary tangles but
not senile (neuritic) plaques in the overlying neocortex in the postmortem brain.
Such white matter lesions, he suggested, might reflect wallerian degeneration of
long corticofugal fiber tracks derived from pyramidal neurons in layer V of the
neocortex, which degenerate with neurofibrillary tangle formation in Alzheimer's
disease.

The Down's syndrome model for Alzheimer's disease is not entirely understood. Wisniewski et al. (1985), among others, showed by cross-sectional postmortem studies that virtually all Down's syndrome patients over the age of 40
years have some Alzheimer neuropathology. However, senile (neuritic) plaques in
the Down's syndrome brain appear to reach their maximum density about 10–20
years before large numbers of neurofibrillary tangles appear. This observation,

and the presentation by Dr. Schapiro that demented older Down's syndrome subjects have reduced cerebral metabolic rates (whereas nondemented older subjects do not have abnormal rates), as well as accelerated ventricular dilatation on CT, led Dr. Schapiro to hypothesize that neuronal loss together with neurofibrillary tangles is necessary (though perhaps not sufficient) for the appearance of dementia in Down's syndrome. A recent paper by Crystal et al. (1988), which analyzes neuropathology in cognitively abnormal patients with and without a diagnosis of Alzheimer's disease, similarly argues that neurofibrillary tangles, with cell loss and progressive atrophy, are required for the appearance of overt dementia in Alzheimer's disease.

Dr. Haxby indicated that hemispheric metabolic asymmetries, a measure of topographic heterogeneity of the disease process, occur frequently in Alzheimer patients and are stable over time in mildly and moderately demented patients. The metabolic asymmetries correlate with appropriate neocortically mediated cognitive abnormalities. Dr. Haxby's additional observation that very early cognitive abnormalities in Alzheimer patients involve memory and directed attention suggests new directions for cognitive stimulation studies in Alzheimer patients, using positron-emission tomograph (PET).

Dr. Rossor also addressed the issue of disease heterogeneity. He discussed a subgroup of patients with primary progressive aphasia, in which reduced blood flow on PET was found routinely in the superior temporal gyrus. Further, he identified a subgroup of Alzheimer patients, or rather "dementia of the Alzheimer type (DAT)" patients, with extrapyramidal signs and who presumably have abnormal central dopaminergic function. However, when using ^{18}F-labeled L-dopa with PET, he could not demonstrate abnormal uptake of tracer within the striatum of these patients, although his research group had reported such abnormal uptake by the putamen of patients with Parkinson's disease. ^{18}F-labeled L-dopa may be a more limited tracer than ^{18}F-labeled 2-deoxy-D-glucose with PET, however, the L-dopa model is less quantitative and more difficult to interpret. Drs. Schapiro and Morrison, commenting on Dr. Rossor's paper, suggested that the extrapyramidal DAT subgroup may have dopaminergic defects in the ventral tegmental area and frontal cortex, areas not explicitly examined by Dr. Rossor in his PET studies. For each Alzheimer subgroup, in any case, it is critical to obtain explicit postmortem information so as to confirm the diagnosis and to relate symptoms to the topography of neuropathology.

Dr. Baron pointed out that, as the brain consists of networks of connected regions which can influence each other, it is not clear, from PET studies alone, whether a reduction in cerebral metabolism or blood flow reflects neuropathology in this region or in another region whose afferent input to the metabolically abnormal region is altered. He based his comments on data that he had gathered on thalamic and striatal infarcts using PET, in which overlying neocortical regions showed transient reductions in brain glucose metabolism. Dr. Baron's proposal that reduced metabolism, even in Alzheimer's disease, could result from "deactivation disconnection" rather than from primary neuropathology, is supported in one case by a report by Dr. Schapiro (1990). In this report, Dr. Schapiro identified a patient who was demented, and who showed the cerebral metabolic abnormalities of DAT prior to death. On postmortem, however, the patient was found to have Parkinson's disease, without obvious neocortical pathology, suggesting that his reduced neocortical metabolism arose from reduced input to the neocortex. Indeed, such examples force us to question the specificity of metabolic and cognitive findings in Alzheimer's disease as compared, for example, with those in reversible depression or the dementia of Parkinson's disease.

Dr. Baron also lamented the dearth of reports which relate regional metabolic or flow abnormalities, measured during life, to regional distribution of neuropathology or regional neurochemistry in the postmortem brain. Thus, we are frequently forced to compare different sets of data from different studies to guess at the basis of the metabolic or flow abnormalities. These might be better understood if metabolism/flow and postmortem pathological measurements were available in the same patient population.

Dr. Paulson also illustrated the topographic heterogeneity of Alzheimer's disease, by his studies of regional cerebral blood flow with single photon emission computed tomography (SPECT). Findings in our laboratory agree with his frequencies of approximately 25% frontal lobe flow deficits, 50% parietal/temporal deficits, and 25% global deficits in Alzheimer patients. These frequencies have been reported by Grady et al. (1989), using the deoxyglucose technique with PET. However, no one appears to understand why the disease may affect one part of the neocortex before another in an individual patient. In this regard, there is the interesting paper by Arendt et al. (1985), who correlated the number and distribution of senile plaques in the neocortex of each cerebral hemisphere with cell loss in appropriate cortical projecting parts of the nucleus basalis of Meynert. Individuals who had more plaques in one than in the other hemisphere also had greater cell loss in the basalis regions which projected to most affected hemisphere.

Dr. Klunk's presentation showed that nuclear magnetic resonance spectroscopy with localization provides a new and appealing method to look at brain intermediary metabolism in relation to other measures of brain function and structure. Regional changes in concentrations of phosphomonoesters and phosphodiesters, as demonstrated with MRI in the Alzheimer brain, provide exciting new evidence for defects in the metabolism of phospholipids, the structural components of cell membranes, and participants in neuronal processes including signal transduction. In this regard, our laboratory has been working on a technique to examine local turnover and synthesis of brain phospholipids in vivo, using radiolabeled fatty acid tracers (Robinson and Rapoport, in press). The method works in animals; perhaps it will find application with PET in humans. After all, much of the brain is lipid. In Alzheimer's disease, cells are dying, and some are trying to recover (Scheibel and Tomayasu 1978; Cotman and Anderson 1988). Thus, it would be informative to look at turnover and synthesis of cell lipid components early in the course of disease and perhaps in relation to drug action.

Many new PET and SPECT techniques are being developed to look at local receptor integrity and number, local blood flow, and various aspects of intermediary metabolism, including protein metabolism. Clearly, we would need another full day at this symposium to consider the potential of these new methodologies for examining the spectrum of brain changes in Alzheimer's disease. Nevertheless, we should be gratified with the presentations and with the conclusions that we have drawn from them. This has been one of the few meetings on Alzheimer's disease which has provided a relatively consistent interpretation of the disease with respect to cerebral topography and its implications. Our plans for studying Alzheimer's disease can now be more rational than those with which we began the symposium.

I thank the Ipsen Foundation for having invited me and the other guests to participate in this exciting program, and I thank the speakers and audience for their creative contributions. This meeting should allow us to obtain appropriate answers – perhaps within only a few years – as to why and how selected brain regions are vulnerable to Alzheimer degeneration.

References

Arendt T, Bigl V, Tennstedt A, Arendt A (1985) Neuronal loss in different parts of the nucleus basalis is related to neuritic plaque formation in cortical target areas in Alzheimer's disease. Neuroscience 14:1–14

Cotman CW, Anderson KJ (1988) Synaptic plasticity and functional stabilization in the hippocampal formation: possible role in Alzheimer's disease. Adv Neurol 47:313–335

Crystal H, Dickson D, Fuld P, Masur D, Scott R, Mehler M, Masdeu J, Kawas C, Aronson M, Wolfson L (1988) Clinico-pathological studies in dementia: nondemented subjects with pathologically confirmed Alzheimer's disease. Neurology 38:1682–1687

Grady CL, Haxby J, Schapiro MB, Kumar A, Friedland RP, Rapoport SI (1989) Heterogeneity in dementia of the Alzheimer type (DAT): subgroups identified from cerebral metabolic patterns using positron emission tomography (PET). Neurology 39 (Suppl 1):167–168

Hyman BT, Van Hoesen GW, Damasio AR, Barnes CL (1984) Alzheimer's disease: cell-specific pathology isolates the hippocampal formation. Science 225:1168–1170

Neve RL, Finch EA, Bird ED, Benowitz LI (1988a) Growth-associated protein GAP-43 is expressed selectively in associative regions of the adult human brain. Proc Natl Acad Sci USA 85:3638–3642

Neve RL, Finch EA, Dawes LR (1988b) Expression of the Alzheimer amyloid precursor gene transcripts in the human brain. Neuron 1:669–677

Robinson PJ, Rapoport SI (in press) A method for examining turnover and synthesis of palmitate-containing brain lipids in vivo. Clin Exp Pharmacol Psychiatry

Schapiro MB, Grady C, Ball MJ, DeCarli C, Rapoport SI (1990) Reductions in parietal/temporal cerebral glucose metabolism are not specific for Alzheimer's disease. Abstr 140 P 42nd Annual Meeting, American Academy Neurology. April 30–May 6, 1990, Miami Beach

Scheibel AB, Tomayasu U (1978) Dendritic sprouting in Alzheimer's presenile dementia. Exp Neurol 60:1–8

Wisniewski KE, Wisniewski HM, Wen GY (1985) Occurrence of neuropathological changes and dementia of Alzheimer's disease in Down's syndrome. Ann Neurol 17:278–282

Subject Index